To the thousands of patients who have trusted us with their most precious sense—their sight.

CATARACT SURGERY

A Patient's Guide to Cataract Treatment

Robert K. Maloney, MD, Inc.

Addicus Books
Omaha, Nebraska

An Addicus Nonfiction Book

ISBN: 978-1-886039-9-40

Illustrations by Bausch & Lomb, Advanced Medical Optics, Mark Erickson, jirehdesign.com, and Jack Kusler.

Typography by Linda Dageforde.

This book is not intended to serve as a substitute for a physician. Nor is it the author's intent to give medical advice contrary to that of an attending physician.

Library of Congress Cataloging-in-Publication Data
Robert K. Maloney, MD, Inc.
　　Cataract surgery : a patient's guide to cataract treatment / Robert K. Maloney, MD, Inc.
　　　p. Cm.
　　Includes bibliographical references and index.
　　ISBN 978-1-886039-94-0 (alk. paper)
　　1. Cataract—Surgery—Popular works. I. Title.

RE451.D48 2008
617.7'42059—dc22　　　　　　　　　　　　　　　　　2008029990

Addicus Books
P.O. Box 45327
Omaha, Nebraska 68145
www.addicusbooks.com

Printed in the United States of America
10　9　8　7　6　5　4　3　2

Contents

Acknowledgments

I wish to thank my father, who taught me to be uncompromising in the pursuit of excellence, and my mother, who taught me that great relationships require compromise. I particularly thank my fabulous wife, Nicole, for her patience with the demands of my chosen career. At times, she must wish that I had listened more to my mother's advice.

—Robert K. Maloney, MD

Introduction

O f all the amazing components of the human anatomy, the eyes may be the most marvelous. They are your primary tools of awareness. The ability to see allows you independence, mobility, and appreciation of visual beauty and form.

If your vision is starting to blur and you think you might have cataracts, put your mind at ease. Cataracts are usually painless, and they are not harmful to other parts of your eyes. They're not a sign of disease, nor are they "growths." They are simply clouding of the lens of the eye.

In most cases, cataracts are as normal a part of aging as the "silver threads among the gold" (in the words of an old song) that appear when your hair begins to gray.

Cataracts develop so gradually that you probably won't need any treatment for them at first. A stronger eyeglass prescription will likely help in the early stages. Eventually, your vision will become blurrier, some things will seem out of focus, and you'll need new prescriptions more often. Objects might appear yellowish. Glare or halos from light sources could make night driving difficult. You might have trouble reading, both close up and at a distance—fine print in a book, for example, and street signs along the highway. When these symptoms interfere with your day-to-day activities, you may want to consider surgery.

By age sixty-five, most Americans have early-stage cataracts, and, by age eighty, most have had cataract surgery. Surgeons perform some 3 million cataract operations a year in the United States, with a very high success rate and few complications.

In many parts of the world, modern cataract surgery is not readily available. Nearly 1 percent of Earth's population is blind, and cataracts cause about half of these cases. Dedicated physicians and public-health professionals regularly donate their time and services to treat cataracts and to purify contaminated water supplies, since parasites are a leading cause of vision loss where fresh, clean water is unavailable.

Thus, we are doubly fortunate to live in a time and a place where outpatient surgery, which takes just minutes, can painlessly replace a clouded natural lens with a state-of-the-art synthetic lens. Within a day or two of your surgery, you'll marvel at how clear and vivid your world has become. And you'll never take your eyesight for granted again.

In the United States, cataract surgery is among the most effective and safest surgical procedures performed—especially in the hands of a highly qualified and experienced eye surgeon. Replacement lenses do an excellent job of restoring vision (with or without glasses, depending on the type of lens implanted). Recovery is rapid—you can resume most of your normal activities within a few days.

This book describes how the healthy eye functions, how cataracts can interfere with clear eyesight, and how clarity can be restored. It explains all your options if cataracts are starting to cloud your vision and it can help you and your doctor determine the right time for surgery.

You, or someone you care about, might find great reassurance in the knowledge that cataracts can be safely and successfully treated and that, once removed, cataracts do not return. Advances in cataract surgery have made it possible for millions of people to enjoy the independence and the aesthetic pleasure of clear vision for decades beyond what was once possible.

The Human Eye and How It Works

To understand how *cataracts* cause blurry vision, you'll probably find it helpful to know something about the structure of the eye and how it works. The eye is a complex organ that performs many complicated functions in a very short time—in the blink of an eye, you might say.

Anatomy of the Eye

If you could examine an entire human eye, you'd see a sphere about an inch in diameter—the size of a large gumball. The eyeball itself is really three thin layers surrounding a fluid-filled center.

Sclera

The outside layer is the "white of the eye," called the *sclera*. It is the tough, opaque tissue that serves as the eye's protective outer coat. Six tiny muscles connect to it around the eye and control the

Anatomy of the Eye

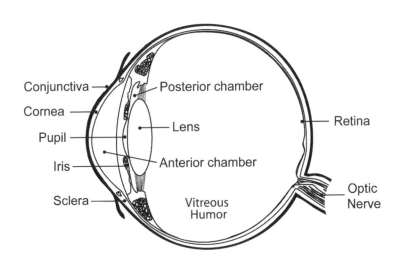

eye's movements. The *optic nerve* is attached to the sclera at the very back of the eye.

Cornea

Curving out from the sclera, the clear *cornea* is the "front window" of the eye. The cornea is amazingly strong and protective against dust and germs. Packed with nerve fibers, it is also quite sensitive to pain. This pain sensitivity is one of the cornea's protective qualities; the pain is a signal that something is trying to invade the eye.

Iris

Under the sclera is another thin layer, which consists of the *iris*—the eye's visible colored ring; when we say that someone's eyes are blue, brown, or green, we are talking about the color of the iris. Besides being an interesting and expressive feature of the face, the iris is essential to clear vision. It surrounds the round, black *pupil*—along with muscle fibers and blood vessels.

Lens

The muscle fibers hold the *lens* of the eye in place and allow it to change its shape so that it can focus on objects at different distances. Located behind the iris and the pupil, the lens is about two-thirds water and one-third protein fibers. There are three distinct layers in the lens, sometimes compared to the layers of a peach:

The *capsule* (the peach "skin") is a thin, clear membrane that forms the outside layer of the lens.

The *cortex* (comparable to the peach "flesh") is the soft, clear material just beneath the capsule.

The *nucleus* (the "pit" of the peach) is the firm center, or core, of the lens.

Retina

The blood vessels, located toward the back of the eye, feed essential nutrients to the *retina,* a smooth, thin layer of nerve tissue at the back of the eye. When you are looking at an object, the retina is where the image comes into focus. Most of the retina contains specialized cells that convert the reflected light (the image) to signals your brain can interpret.

The *macula* is the focal point at the center of the retina. Within the macula are millions of light-sensitive nerve endings that act as *photoreceptors.*

The photoreceptors called *rods* are sensitive to brightness and allow us to see in dim light.

The photoreceptors called *cones* respond to the varying wavelengths of light that produce different colors.

The *fovea centralis,* in the center of the macula, is densely packed with cone cells. It is the fovea that gives your eye the ability to sharpen an image. The clearest vision—what we call "*20/20 vision*"—would be impossible without the fovea.

Another part of the retina, the *retinal pigment epithelium,* consists of dark tissue cells that absorb excess light and carry nutrients to, and waste products from, the retina.

Features that Protect the Eyes

The eyeballs are protected, in part, by their location—they are embedded in *sockets,* which are strongholds of bone, fat, and muscle. Other protective features of the eye are:

- *Eyelashes,* which protect your eyes from dust, contaminants, and other small particles

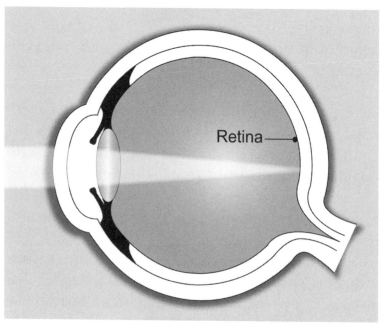

Retina

The lens is clear in this normal eye, allowing light to pass through.

- *Eyebrows,* which trap liquids (such as perspiration) and particles that might otherwise find their way into your eyes
- *Tears,* which supply moisture that not only keeps your eyes from drying out but also contain substances that fight bacteria. If a foreign object gets into your eye, tear production increases to flush it out. When perspiration drips into your eyes, the high salt content makes your eyes sting, and the stinging stimulates tear production. The tears dilute the salty perspiration (or other liquid

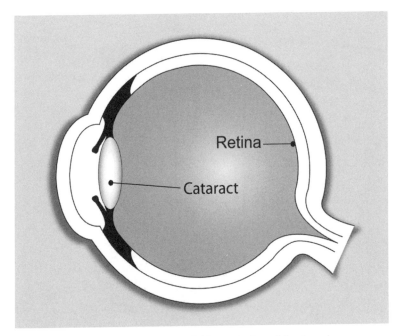

A cataract has formed in the lens of this eyeball, and the lens has become cloudy.

that might accidentally enter your eye) and cleanse the eye.

- *Eyelids,* which work like windshield wipers when you blink, to spread tears across the cornea. Blinking is usually automatic—you seldom have to remember to blink—but it is also a protective reflex that goes into action when your eyes perceive an object moving toward them or are assaulted by extremely bright light.

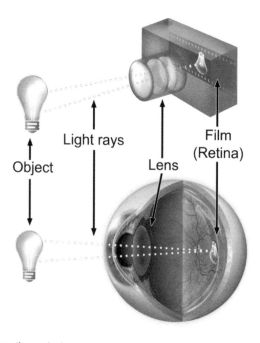

Light passes through the eyeball lens and lands on the retina in the same way light passes through a camera lens and on to the film.

How Vision Occurs

Let's say you're looking at autumn leaves. Light reflects off the leaves and enters the eye through the cornea, then travels through several structures to the back of the eye, where the image reaches its sharpest focus. From there, the optic nerve carries the focused "leaves images" to the brain. Only then can you actually see the leaves.

Let's take a closer look at this process. It might be helpful to think of seeing as four distinct processes, which are roughly similar to the way a camera processes an image.

1. Light Reflects Off an Object

When you're admiring the beautiful orange and red foliage on a maple tree in autumn, you're actually seeing the light reflecting off them—just as a photograph is an image of light reflecting off an object. If this were not the case, then you'd be able to see objects at night, or photograph them, just as well as in daylight.

2. Light Enters the Eye

As it reaches the eye, the form of energy that we call *light* first enters the clear, curved cornea. The curved surface of the cornea bends the incoming light so that the rays come together, like branches, instead of remaining parallel as they enter the eye. Thus the cornea does most of the focusing work of the eye.

After passing through the cornea, light is bathed in a thin layer of liquid, the *aqueous humor,* before it reaches the iris. The iris contracts or expands *(dilates)* around the pupil to regulate the amount of light allowed into the eye's interior. Sophisticated cameras have light-regulating mechanisms that do much the same thing.

When you walk out of a dark movie theater into bright daylight, you've probably experienced that "blinding" sensation before the iris has time to contract, adjusting to the difference in light.

3. Light Is Focused in the Lens

The lens, by changing its shape, also contributes to the eye's focusing work. The lens is round and usually somewhat flat. When you were younger, most likely your eye lenses were perfectly clear and quite flexible. Some eye specialists compare the lens to a small, clear gelcap with a thin but sturdy exterior. If you squeeze it in the middle, it gets thinner and flatter; if you squeeze the ends, it gets thicker and more rounded.

That's basically what happens to the eye lens when you focus on objects at varying distances, except that the work of "squeezing," or contracting, is done by muscles called *ciliary muscles* and the ligaments attached to them (*zonules*). These muscles and ligaments also hold the lens in place.

When you focus on something close up, the ciliary muscles contract, making the lens thicker and rounder. As your focus moves outward to more-distant objects, the muscles relax and the lens becomes thinner and flatter. Thus, the lens projects a clear image onto the retina, at the back of the eye, whether the source of the image is near or far, or somewhere between.

This shape-changing adjustment to distance is called *accommodation*. Although the cornea does the initial focusing, it is the lens and its accommodation ability that allow you to focus well at different distances.

Once light passes through the lens, it enters the spacious cavity that occupies about two-thirds of the eye. This cavity is filled with a clear gel called *vitreous,* or *vitreous humor,* which helps the eye maintain its round shape.

4. Light Signals Are Interpreted by the Brain

Finally, the light reaches its destination—the retina, which receives images in much the same way that camera film does. After the retina's specialized cells, rods, and cones have converted the image to signals that the brain can understand, the signals are finally carried to the brain through the nerve bundle at the back of eye—the optic nerve, which consists of millions of nerve fibers. The brain receives and interprets the signals, and it is at that point that we actually see.

The eye is sometimes described as an extension of the brain, and if there is severe damage to the optic nerve, the eye becomes useless. Vision occurs only when an image reaches the brain and is identified.

Eye-Structure Abnormalities

The process described above works best if the eye is a perfect sphere and the cornea is smooth and rounded. Often this isn't the case. The eye might be shorter or longer from front to back than it is from top to bottom, or the cornea's curvature might be slightly flattened.

Hyperopia

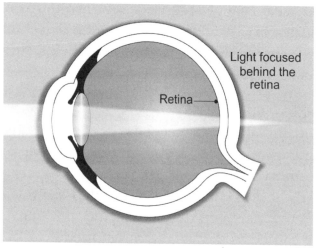

Also called farsightedness, hyperopia causes light rays to focus behind the retina. Objects in the distance are seen more clearly than those up close.

Astigmatism

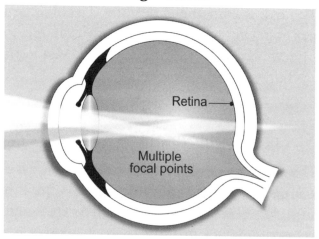

Astigmatism causes objects both far and near to appear blurry, because a curvature in the cornea prevents light rays from uniformly focusing on the retina.

Myopia

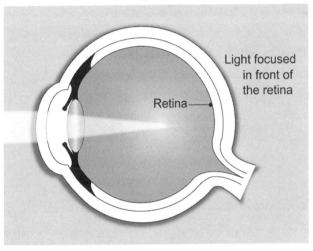

Also known as being nearsighted, myopia causes distant images to appear blurry because images focus in front of the retina rather than on it.

Farsightedness and Nearsightedness

If your own eyes are shorter than normal from front to back, then you have *hyperopia,* or *farsightedness,* and you see distant objects more clearly than near ones. If the opposite is true—your eyes are too long from front to back—you have *myopia,* or *nearsightedness,* and you have trouble seeing distant objects.

Astigmatism

The cornea's curvature should be rounded, like the side of a basketball. If, instead, it's shaped more like the side of a football, it will produce two focal points instead of just one. This condition is called

15

astigmatism and it causes blur and distortion, especially up close.

Cataracts and Lens Function

You can see how many structures and processes are important to the act of seeing. If just one structure is defective or one process doesn't work properly, the eyesight—so important to most of us in almost everything we do—can be damaged. Like other parts of our bodies, our eyes don't function as well when we age as they did when we were young.

Cataracts are the most common age-related eye defect. The next chapter will explain what cataracts are and how they interfere with the intricate function of the lens.

2

What Is a Cataract?

If you're in your mid-fifties or older, there's a good chance that your eyes have started to develop cataracts. You can't see them, you can't feel them, and until they begin to seriously affect your vision you don't really need to do anything about them except continue to take good care of your eyes. That means having regular eye exams and protecting your eyes—from injury, from the sun's *ultraviolet* (UV) rays, and from irritants such as dust and wind.

A cataract is a clouding of the natural lens inside the eye. The clouded areas are often called *opacities* because they are opaque, meaning they are not clear, and light cannot pass through. The lens must be crystal clear to do its focusing job, so the areas of opacity interfere with good vision.

What Causes Cataracts?

Protein fibers in the lens, called *crystallines*, are precisely arranged in thousands of layers. Usually because of aging, the proteins deteriorate or become "disarranged." Some scientists believe that these fragmented proteins cause the densities, or "clumps," that cloud areas of the lens. These dense areas are cataracts, and as they become larger they cause noticeable vision loss.

People sometimes confuse cataracts with an unrelated lens condition, *presbyopia*—a stiffening of the lens also caused by aging. Throughout life, the lens continues to manufacture new layers of cells, and the accumulation of layers makes the lens less pliable. As the lens loses its flexibility, it also loses the ability to accommodate as well as it once could.

Normal Eye

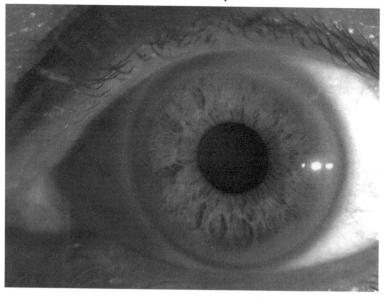

This is a normal eye. Note the clarity of the lens.

At about age forty-five, most people—even those who have had excellent vision—find that "their arms are too short." They have to hold books and magazines farther from their eyes in order to focus on the print. If presbyopia is your only vision problem, you can probably solve it with inexpensive reading glasses.

Types of Cataracts

You will usually see cataracts classified according to their location on the lens: *nuclear, cortical,* or *subcapsular.* A nuclear cataract is the most common and is the type most associated with aging, although older patients often have more than one type.

Nuclear Cataracts

A nuclear cataract, as the name suggests, is a clouding of the *center* of the lens, almost always due to aging. One of the early symptoms, oddly enough, is that your near vision will improve for a while. This improvement, referred to as *second sight,* is short-lived, however. As the cataract advances, the lens becomes yellow or even brown. Vision becomes dimmer and blurrier, and you're likely to have trouble distinguishing colors. *Glare* might bother you, making it hard to drive at night. You may need stronger light for pursuits such as reading and needlework.

Nuclear Cataract

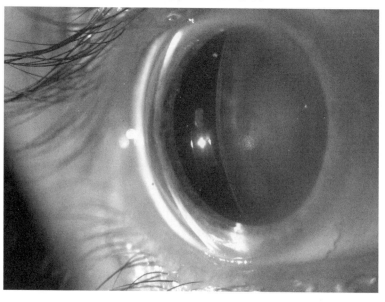

Nuclear cataracts are the most common type of cataract. Usually caused by aging, they typically cloud the center of the lens.

Cortical Cataracts

Many people develop cortical cataracts with age. These cataracts begin as whitish, wedge-shaped opaque areas on the outer edge of the lens cortex, near the capsule. Slowly, these opacities become streaks reaching inward to the center of the lens, like spokes on a wheel. When they reach the center, they block part of the light passing through the nucleus of the lens, and you will begin to have problems with focusing, distortion, and glare. Because both distance and near vision are impaired, you may require surgery at a comparatively early

Cortical Cataract

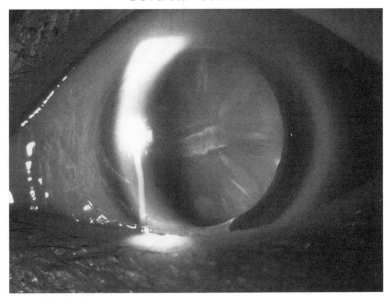

The second most common cataract, a cortical cataract forms as a wedge on the outside of the lens and gradually extends "spokes" to the center of the lens.

stage. If you have diabetes, you may be particularly susceptible to cortical cataracts.

Subcapsular Cataracts

When a subcapsular cataract begins at the back of the lens, which is most often the case, it's called a *posterior subcapsular cataract.* It starts out as a grainlike opaque area under the lens capsule. Because posterior subcapsular cataracts are usually directly in the path of light on its way to the retina,

Subcapsular Cataract

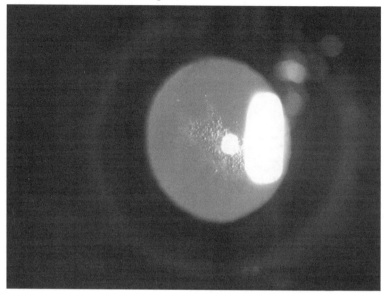

Subcapsular cataracts form at the back of the lens and block light, causing vision problems.

you might have vision problems early on, particularly with glare and *halos*.

Anyone can have subcapsular cataracts in one or both eyes. People who are extremely nearsighted, who have diabetes, or who are taking high doses of *steroids* are particularly at risk.

How Common Are Cataracts?

Nearly everyone will eventually have cataracts. Estimates differ because not all who are affected seek treatment, but current research indicates that by age seventy-five at least 70 percent of Americans either have had cataract surgery or cannot see well because of cataracts. You'll likely begin to notice cataract-related vision problems in your early to mid-sixties.

Cataract surgery is the most common surgical procedure in the United States. Some 3 million Americans have cataract surgery every year, often in an outpatient procedure that takes less than ten to fifteen minutes. The surgeon replaces the clouded natural lens with a clear synthetic lens through a tiny incision. These procedures nearly always succeed in greatly improving the patient's vision, with almost no interruption in daily activities.

How Do Cataracts Affect the Eyes?

As explained earlier, all light entering the eye passes through the lens. Your lens must be clear for light to focus properly on the retina. Therefore, any clouding of the lens will affect your vision to some extent.

In most people, cataracts develop gradually and their eyesight may be adequate for several years before surgery is necessary. Other people experience more-rapid progression of cataracts, especially if several areas of the lens are affected. Cataracts that form directly behind the pupil are likely to cause problems sooner than cataracts closer to the edges of the lens.

As more and more of the lens becomes opaque, the clouded areas scatter the light that enters and prevent it from focusing properly on the retina. If you have cataracts, sensitivity to glare might make it hard to drive at night. You might see halos around lights. Your vision might be blurred or hazy—like trying to see through a waterfall. (In fact, it might be that sensation that gave cataracts their name: The Latin term for "waterfall" is *cataracta.* Another theory is that the whitish color of an eye cataract is similar to the color of turbulent water, as in a waterfall.)

Eventually, the lens takes on a yellow or brown tinge, which affects your ability to distinguish colors, particularly shades of purple and blue. Again, these changes might occur so slowly that you don't notice them until someone points out that your socks don't match!

Age-related cataracts don't spread from one eye to the other, though they typically develop at about the same rate in both eyes. Cataracts, if neglected, can advance to the point where the pupils appear milky. These cataracts are referred to as *ripe* or *mature.* (At one time, patients were advised to wait until their cataracts were ripe before having surgery. This approach was abandoned long ago.)

Immature cataracts, in which there are still clear areas of the lens, are generally not visible except to the doctor who is examining your eyes. You would almost surely notice significant vision changes and seek treatment long before your cataracts were ripe and visible to the naked eye.

Unless they are persistently ignored and become *overripe,* cataracts do *not* cause discomfort—itching, burning, or aching—or a discharge from your eye, nor do they create redness, swelling, or inflammation. If you have symptoms such as these, see your eye doctor to find out what *is* causing them.

Can Cataracts Cause Blindness?

With continued neglect, a cataract may turn completely white and become painful and inflamed. Described as overripe or *hypermature,* these cataracts are so advanced that the patient has little or no vision in the affected eye. Surgery is essential to remove the inflamed lens. This surgery is more difficult and recovery takes longer than the usual lens-replacement procedure.

Only if you ignore them and fail to get proper treatment are cataracts likely to cause blindness. Many people, unfortunately, do not receive treatment, which is why cataracts are the most common cause of blindness worldwide.

There are a variety of reasons that cataracts go untreated: In some parts of the world, safe and effective cataract surgery is not readily available. Even in the United States and other developed nations, however, many people are afraid to see a doctor about their failing vision. Some of them fear surgery, not realizing that lens replacement is a quick and virtually painless outpatient procedure with a very high success rate.

We've touched on signs and symptoms of cataracts. The next chapter will discuss these symptoms in greater detail and will help you and your doctor decide when it's time to consider surgery for your cataracts.

3

Signs and Symptoms

You've been wearing the same pair of glasses for years. You go in for your regular eye exam, and your eye doctor gives you a stronger prescription. Six months later, you're back, complaining that your new prescription is already too weak. The first sign of cataracts is often the need for more-frequent prescriptions. A cataract might develop earlier in one eye than the other, but both eyes will eventually be affected.

Cataracts Symptoms

Not all cataracts produce the same symptoms. The type of cataract you have will determine the type of symptoms you may notice.

Clouded, Blurred, or Dim Vision

Cataracts on any part of the lens can cause fuzzy vision, but posterior subcapsular cataracts are likely to do so earlier in their development, as mentioned. As you'll recall from chapter 2, a posterior subcapsular cataract is located just beneath the capsule at the back of the eye, near the retina, where the area of incoming light is smallest. The cataract might not be very big, but it obstructs the cone of light at its narrowest point.

Nuclear cataracts, at the center of the eye, are directly in the path of incoming light. At first, nuclear cataracts, being thicker than the natural lens, might act like a magnifying glass, making close-up objects clearer. This short-term improvement in near vision, called second sight, is lost as the cataract worsens.

Halos and Glare

Bigger pupils create a larger pathway for light entering the eye, so more of the lens—including the edges of cortical and subcapsular cataracts—is exposed. When sudden bright light—car headlights, even street lighting and stoplights—enters the eye, the exposed cataract edges "scatter" it, causing halos and glare. A halo is a circle of light around a light source. Glare is light that dazzles and seems almost blindingly bright.

You've experienced this scattering of light when you've driven at night with a fogged-up windshield. The tiny drops of moisture on the window bend the incoming light in multiple directions, nearly blinding you with glare and making it very difficult to see where you're going.

Sensitivity to glare can occur with all types of cataracts. In general, glare is less troublesome for people with nuclear cataracts than for those with cortical cataracts. Posterior subcapsular cataracts usually produce the worst glare.

Some people find glare to be not only inconvenient but almost painful. If cataracts are making you extremely sensitive to glare and interfering with your day-to-day activities, discuss the possibility of surgery with your eye doctor.

Loss of Contrast

Scattering of light inside the eye also causes *loss of contrast,* making it hard for you to distinguish the edges of dark objects alongside lighter-colored ones. You might not be able to clearly see black lettering on a white page, or trees silhouetted against a bright sky.

Ghost Images and Double Vision

The tendency of cataracts to scatter light entering the lens can also cause *double vision,* especially if you're looking at a light source. *Ghost images* are similar to "seeing double." With double vision, however, you'll see two relatively clear images, whereas ghost images are fainter "copies" that appear on one side of or around the object you're looking at.

Just as we are either right-handed or left-handed, we also have a dominant eye. Ghost images and double vision usually affect the dominant eye more than the weaker one.

Difficulty Seeing in Bright Light

In bright light the pupil becomes smaller, narrowing the pathway through which light enters the eye. A nuclear cataract located in that pathway is more likely to obstruct your vision when your pupils are constricted and the pathway is narrow.

Change in Color Vision

Age-related cataracts become grayish or yellowish as they thicken. Naturally, these tints affect your ability to distinguish colors. It's common for people with cataracts to report that colors look washed-out, faded, or yellowish.

Dealing with Early Cataract Symptoms

In cataracts' early stages, getting stronger glasses or contacts and using a magnifying glass, a page magnifier, or better lighting can help you see more clearly. The American Foundation for the Blind recommends the following light sources for people with cataracts:

- *Sunlight*—but use proper eye protection if outside, and use window treatments if inside. Wear a hat with a visor or ultraviolet-filtering sunglasses outdoors. Indoors, reduce glare by sitting with your back to the window and by using window tinting, lattices, adjustable blinds, or sheer curtains.

- *Full-spectrum or warm fluorescent bulbs* can produce strong light and have several advantages over incandescent lights: They don't burn as hot, they don't create shadows, they last longer, and they use less energy. Many stores that sell fluorescent bulbs take back the burned-out ones for proper disposal. Call your local recycling center for information on how to dispose of regular and compact fluorescent bulbs.

- *Incandescent bulbs* have few advantages, now that miniature fluorescents are available for lamps. Incandescents do emit steady, constant light, whereas fluorescent bulbs may flicker, especially when they are about to burn out, and the flickering might be bothersome for some people with cataracts. If you're buying incandescent bulbs, look for those labeled "full-spectrum," which simulate natural sunlight.

- *Halogen bulbs* are more energy efficient than incandescents, but they burn hotter. There is some evidence that the amount of blue light that halogen bulbs produce can be harmful to the eyes, and they pose slightly more fire danger than other bulbs.

Experiment with a mix of different types of bulbs to see what works best for you.

Though cataracts are considered a normal consequence of aging, certain lifestyle, environmental, and health factors can cause cataracts to develop earlier—and in different parts of the lens—for some people than for others. We'll examine these factors in the next chapter.

4

Causes and Risk Factors

Although it's true that aging is the number-one risk factor for cataracts, we don't all age at the same rate. If you've taken good care of yourself, your *chronological age*, in years, might be somewhat higher than your *biological age*—measured by the condition of your muscles, brain, lungs, and sensory organs. So what we call aging is, in part, the cumulative effect of damage to the body caused by sun exposure, disease, environment, and a number of other factors.

A lifetime of good health habits probably won't prevent cataracts altogether. If you've been kind to your body, however, it's quite possible that cataracts will develop later and will be less extensive—confined to the nucleus, perhaps, rather than developing in the cortex or the subcapsular area, or both. On the other hand, people with high blood pressure or obesity tend to develop posterior subcapsular cataracts, and taking a thyroid hormone may contribute to cortical-cataract development.

How Aging Takes a Toll

When aging takes its toll early, *free radicals* might be to blame. Free radicals are atoms, usually oxygen, that have an odd number of electrons, leaving one electron unpaired. This *free electron* makes the atom unstable, so it "seeks out" other particles in the body to bond with.

Excess free radicals steal electrons from normal particles in other cells, damaging their DNA and converting *them* to free radicals. The mutated cells multiply abnormally and rapidly, creating a chain reaction. Rampant free-radical damage is a factor in accelerated aging as well as dozens of disorders, including cancer, heart disease, strokes, emphysema, diabetes, rheumatoid arthritis, osteoporosis, ulcers, Crohn's disease, Alzheimer's disease, Parkinson's disease...and cataracts.

What produces free-radical overload? There are at least four lifestyle factors that aggravate free-radical damage:

1. The body's overproduction of free radicals, caused by tobacco use (not only smoking but also using snuff or chewing tobacco), air pollution, certain disease processes, poisons, drugs, radiation (ultraviolet light, X-rays, and gamma rays from radioactive material), polyunsaturated and hydrogenated oils, rancid fats and nuts, smoked

and barbecued foods, some food additives, and other substances

2. Undernourishment, producing too few of the *antioxidants* needed to fight free radicals

3. Activities and substances that affect metabolism, causing the body to use up its supply of antioxidants too quickly (stress, "extreme" exercise, certain illnesses, obesity, drugs, and toxins)

4. Alcohol abuse, which not only consumes more than its share of antioxidants but also is believed to act directly on lens proteins

Free radicals aren't all bad. It's normal for cells, during the process of creating energy, to produce free radicals. Sometimes, however, our bodies produce more free radicals than our antioxidant supply can soak up. Antioxidants such as vitamins C and E are able to bond with and neutralize these unstable particles.

Nutrition and Free Radicals

You can see why nutrition is so important to long-term wellness. A healthful diet *excludes* substances that create free radicals and *includes* antioxidants, which are present in plants (and plant-eating animals). Supplements containing the recommended amounts of antioxidants such as vitamins C and E, beta-carotene (a form of vitamin

A), selenium, lutein, lycopene, and bioflavonoids may be helpful, but it's better to get your antioxidants from real food.

Here's why: It's not necessarily isolated antioxidants, such as vitamins A and E, that prevent free-radical damage; it's the way these antioxidants are balanced and combined with enzymes, phytonutrients, and other food compounds, helping your body absorb them naturally and conferring the greatest benefits.

Another reason not to depend too heavily on supplements is uncertainty about *bioavailability* and dosage. The term "bioavailability" refers to how readily your body absorbs and uses the compounds contained in supplements. You might already know that too much vitamin A can be fatal. What you might not realize is that other supplements—taken in excess or in a form with low bioavailability—can actually *stimulate* free-radical production rather than *neutralize* free radicals. The combination of nutrients and other compounds in food works to safely regulate your body's absorption of antioxidants.

Antioxidant-Rich Foods
Fruits and Vegetables

With some exceptions (cabbage, cantaloupe, cauliflower, and white potatoes, for example, which are also rich in these beneficial compounds, the more colorful the food, the richer its supply of antioxidants. Color variety is the key to supplying

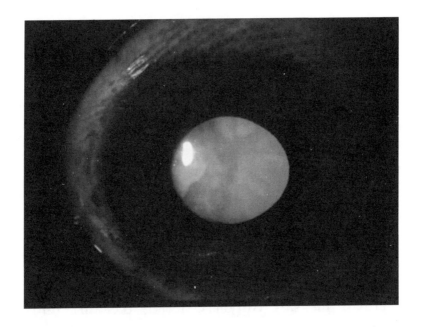

This is an example of a severe nuclear cataract, in which the lens has become totally opaque.

your body with the many beneficial combinations of free-radical-fighting substances.

Antioxidant-rich fruits include blackberries, blueberries, cantaloupe, cherries, cranberries, grapefruit, grapes, pears, plums, raspberries, strawberries, and tomatoes.

Vegetables that are high in antioxidants include garlic, onions, sweet peppers (all colors), carrots, broccoli, beets, potatoes (yams are especially healthful), asparagus, cabbage, cauliflower, and spinach and other dark-green leafy vegetables.

Other Sources of Antioxidants

- Beans, peas, and peanuts

- Olive oil and flaxseed oil
- Whole grains, wheat germ, bran,
- Fish and poultry
- Nuts
- Bee pollen, dark chocolate, green tea, red wine

Go light on salt and sugar, which deplete your body's supply of antioxidants.

Congenital Cataracts

In rare cases, babies are born with cataracts. Mothers used to be concerned about getting German measles (rubella) during the first three months of pregnancy, since the disease could cause birth defects, including cataracts. Fortunately, now that children are routinely vaccinated against rubella, this risk has virtually disappeared in the United States. Other infections and certain medications early in pregnancy can still cause *congenital cataracts,* as can hereditary conditions. These cataracts might or might not cause vision problems. If they do, they are surgically treated in much the same way as are cataracts in adults.

Illness-Related Cataracts

Diabetes mellitus is probably the most highly publicized source of cataracts that form due to disease. People with higher-than-normal blood-sugar

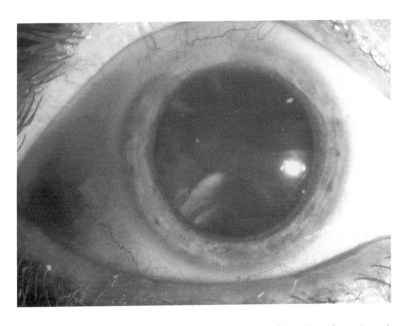

This is an example of a cortical cataract. Vision is affected as the cataract reaches the center of the lens, causing glare and loss of contrast.

levels, even if they are not diabetic, are also at risk for cataracts.

There are dozens of other illnesses that can lead to cataract formation, including hypertension and thyroid disorders.

Traumatic Cataracts

Eye injuries, caused by sharp objects or a direct blow to the eye, can cause *traumatic cataracts.* Traumatic cataracts may also form as a result of a head injury near the eye, earlier eye surgery, eye inflammation, chemical burns, and electric shock.

Some scientists consider radiation a form of "slow trauma" that contributes to cataract development. Overexposure to radiation can come from numerous sources, including:

- Sunlight (ultraviolet light), which is most intense at the equator and accounts for a higher incidence of cataracts among inhabitants of lower latitudes. (Researchers expect this problem to worsen with continued depletion of the ozone layer.)
- Cosmic radiation, which particularly affects commercial airline pilots and astronauts
- Infrared (heat) radiation, usually as a result of prolonged occupational exposure (by glass-blowers, for example—hence the term *glass-blower's cataract*)
- Intense artificial light, such as that used in arc welding
- Radiation therapy near the eye

Other Risk Factors

- Long-term drug use, including chemotherapy and the use of corticosteroids, whether taken orally, inhaled, injected, or applied to the skin
- Heredity; a family history of early cataract development
- Dark eye color

- Gender (women, especially those who started menstruating late, being at higher risk)
- Severe myopia—although eyeglasses, worn for many years, apparently provide protection against ultraviolet radiation and can offset the risk from nearsightedness

Low cholesterol levels in the lens and cerebral cortex can contribute to cataract formation, according to a Japanese study published in 2006. The study cautioned physicians to be aware of this effect when prescribing cholesterol-lowering drugs. Paradoxically, a University of Wisconsin study (2006) and two Australian studies (2007) have shown that taking cholesterol-reducing drugs known as *statins* significantly slows cataract development and also reduces the risk of *macular degeneration.* Researchers are working to clarify the relationship between cholesterol and cataracts.

Can you prevent cataracts? Not entirely. But you might well delay the onset of cataracts by being sensible about sun exposure, wearing UV-protective sunglasses and a hat with a brim when you're outdoors, eating well, keeping fit, learning to relax, and staying upbeat in the face of stress. Delaying cataract formation is just one of many reasons to cultivate a lifestyle that promotes health and well-being.

5

Your Eye Examination

Optics is one of the most advanced fields of scientific research and application. Eye doctors can use amazingly sophisticated machines to examine your eyes microscopically, detecting even the abnormal proteins that are present in cataracts.

Chances are, though, that the first thing you'll do at your eye exam is look at a good old-fashioned eye chart—the same kind eye doctors have been using since the mid-eighteenth century.

Having you read the letters on the eye chart—the *visual acuity test*—is one of the ways your doctor checks for signs of cataracts. For a definite diagnosis, the doctor will use eye drops to dilate your pupils. The wider the pupil, the better he or she can use special lights to examine the inside of the eye and actually see cataracts on the lens.

The various tests described in this chapter give you and your doctor information about the overall health of your eye and about other conditions that might be affecting your eyesight. The tests can reveal how much of your vision loss is due to cataracts rather than, for example, presbyopia, myopia, or eye disease.

Choosing Your Eye Doctor

In the United States, comprehensive eye exams can be performed by *ophthalmologists* and *optometrists*. What's the difference between these specialists?

An ophthalmologist is a medical doctor (MD), like an orthopedic surgeon, neurosurgeon, or plastic surgeon, who has completed medical school, an internship, and an ophthalmology residency to learn the medicine and surgery of the eyes, eyelids, and ocular system. *Cataract and refractive surgeons* are ophthalmologists who further specialize in surgical correction of vision and focusing problems.

An optometrist, also called an optometric doctor (O.D.), specializes in primary eye care including vision correction and medical conditions of the eye. Optometrists can prescribe glasses, contact lenses, and medications, but they do not perform surgery. If an optometrist diagnoses cataracts or eye disease, he or she will refer the patient to an ophthalmologist for treatment. Many optometrists work closely with ophthalmologists to comanage the preoperative and postoperative care of cataract-surgery patients.

An *optician* fits and dispenses eyeglasses and, in some states, contact lenses. Outside the United

States, some countries license *ophthalmic opticians* to perform eye exams.

Who Performs Cataract Surgery?

The surgical treatment of cataracts should be done by an ophthalmologist—one who is well qualified, experienced, and respected by colleagues and patients. You can find out about a doctor's credentials from his or her office, the local medical society, a hospital where the doctor is on staff, or the HMO, if applicable. Several sources on the Internet give you access to national and state sources of physician information.

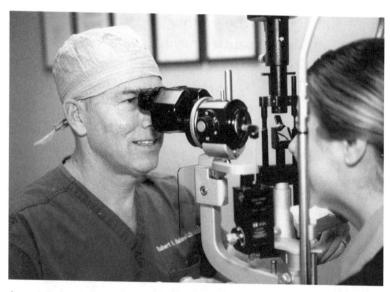

An ophthalmologist uses a slit lamp to perform a microscopic evaluation of the interior of the eyes and to assess the degree of cataract formation.

Ask your optometrist or primary-care physician to recommend an ophthalmologist. If you have cataracts, consider seeking an ophthalmologist who specializes in treating cataracts. If you're leaning toward a particular doctor, arrange to talk with a few of his or her patients. Since cataract surgery is so common, you should have no trouble finding people who have had the procedure.

Scheduling Your Eye Exam

Even if your vision is perfect, you should have a baseline eye exam at age forty, according to the American Academy of Ophthalmology. Your eye doctor can detect even small changes in your vision and eye health by comparing later eye-exam results to the baseline exam.

Don't wait until you're forty if you have diabetes or high blood pressure, if you are taking steroids, if you have a family history of eye disorders, or if you're having problems with your eyes. Schedule your baseline exam right away.

After doing your baseline exam, the doctor will let you know when you should come back. The American Academy of Ophthalmology's recommended eye-exam schedule is:

- every two to four years until you're sixty-five
- every one or two years after age sixty-five
- any time you're having problems with your eyes

Preparing for Your Eye Exam

Before you go to your appointment, assemble your medical records. Your eye doctor will want information about:

- any past eye disorders, injuries, and operations
- past and present medical problems
- all medications you're taking, including contraceptives and other prescription drugs, over-the-counter medications, herbs, and homeopathic products, as well as food supplements such as vitamins and minerals
- any family history of eye disease
- your occupation and hobbies (in order to determine the potential for injury and also to understand how you use your eyes—primarily for driving or computer work, for example)
- your primary-care doctor's name, address, and phone number

Be sure to take your eyeglasses or contact lenses to your appointment. Take sunglasses, too, because your doctor will probably use eye drops to dilate your pupils, and the enlarged pupils will make your eyes extremely sensitive to bright light for several hours. In fact, you might want to arrange for someone to drive you home.

Comprehensive Eye Examination

Your appointment could be as brief as half an hour, but it will more likely require an hour or longer. The length of your exam depends on several factors: What is the doctor looking for? Which, among the dozens of tests available, will be used? In a routine comprehensive exam, the doctor will probably check your eyes for:

- *myopia* (nearsightedness; seeing near objects better than far objects)
- *hyperopia* (farsightedness; seeing distant objects more clearly than near ones)
- *presbyopia* (a form of farsightedness that begins at age forty to forty-five)
- *astigmatism* (irregular lens shape that distorts your vision slightly)
- *strabismus* (*"cross-eye"*) and *amblyopia* (*"lazy eye"*)
- *glaucoma* (high fluid pressure within the eye)
- cataracts, *color blindness,* blocked tear ducts, eye injury, defects on the cornea, and damage to the retina or optic nerve

Visual Acuity Test

A test for visual acuity refers to the clarity of your vision. (*Acuity* is from the Latin *acuitas,* which means "sharpness.") In other words, how well do you see?

Your eye doctor will probably use the familiar eye chart to test your vision at various distances. The eye chart most of us know is called *Snellen's chart*, after the nineteenth-century Dutch ophthalmologist Hermann Snellen, who invented it. It consists of rows of black letters—very large at the top, very small at the bottom—against a white background. Each eye will be tested separately while the other eye is covered. If you've had a problem with glare, the doctor will probably test your visual acuity using a variety of lighting sources.

The results of your visual acuity test are expressed by phrases such as "20/20 vision" and "20/40 vision," which some people find confusing. The first number in the phrase, in the United States at least, is always 20—which is the distance, in feet, you're standing from the eye chart. (Where the metric system is used, the first number is 6, indicating that the patient is standing 6 meters from the chart.)

The second number conveys how much your visual acuity differs from "normal" eyesight. If you have 20/20 vision, you can see at 20 feet what other people with good vision can see at 20 feet. If your vision is 20/40, you can see at 20 feet what people with good vision can see at 40 feet. The higher the second number, the worse your visual acuity. If your vision is 20/70 or worse, you have *low vision*. At

20/200—meaning that someone with "normal" vision standing 200 feet away can see the chart as well as you can at 20 feet away—you are considered *legally blind.* (Only about 10 percent of legally blind Americans have zero visual acuity; the rest have some degree of sight.)

Eye-Movement Examination and Cover Tests

There are other low-tech procedures that are probably familiar to you. These tests don't require fancy equipment, but they give the doctor a lot of important information, including whether you have cross-eye or lazy eye and how good your depth perception is.

He or she will ask you to look upward and downward, and to the right and the left. Then you'll be asked to stare at an object—first at a distance and later up close. The doctor will cover one of your eyes and quickly note how much the uncovered eye moves to adjust, then repeat the process with the other eye. He or she will probably hold an object, perhaps a pencil, near your eyes and ask you to "follow" it as it moves from side to side.

Iris and Pupil Examination

The doctor will check the appearance of the iris. Is it symmetrical? Does the pupil respond correctly to light, dilating and constricting as needed? What is the size of the pupils?

Refractive Error

If your vision is worse than 20/20, the doctor will perform a variety of tests to determine the *correction* needed—that is, to come up with an accurate prescription for eyeglasses or contact lenses.

The degree of farsightedness, nearsightedness, astigmatism, or presbyopia is called *refractive error*. To measure refractive error precisely, the doctor will probably use another rather old-fashioned device called a *phoropter*.

If you've had an eye exam, you're probably familiar with a phoropter. It is a complete range of corrective lenses that can be adjusted to offer you hundreds of combinations. The doctor adjusts the lenses and asks you to indicate which of two combinations is better. By continually changing the lenses, the doctor can arrive at a combination of lens strengths that will be the basis of your prescription.

Though there are automated devices for testing refractive error, many eye doctors report getting the best results by using them in conjunction with the more-subjective phoropter. An *autorefractor* emits a pinpoint beam of light that reflects off the retina and measures the eye's response. Autorefractors are especially useful when the patient is a small child or, perhaps, an adult who is unable to respond accurately to phoropter combinations. Some ophthalmologists use advanced computerized equipment, such as a high-tech scanner called a *wavefront aberrometer,* for more-detailed results.

Dilating the Pupils

For certain additional tests—to examine your general eye health and the retina, optic nerve, and blood vessels—the doctor will need to dilate your pupils using eye drops. These drops take about twenty minutes to fully open the pupils, giving the doctor a much wider view of the inside of your eyes than would be possible with constricted pupils.

After *dilation,* your vision might be blurred and highly sensitive to light for several hours. You won't want to walk out into bright sunlight with your eyes uncovered. If you don't have sunglasses, most eye doctors will give you disposable sunglasses to wear on the way home. Since there's no way of knowing how long it will take your eyes to return to normal, the best course is to arrange for someone to drive you home.

Ophthalmoscopic Examination

An *ophthalmoscope* is a specialized device through which your doctor can inspect the blood vessels and the optic nerve at the back of the eye. He or she will also examine the retina for detachment and tears, and the small areas on the retina responsible for sharp vision (the fovea) and *central vision* (the macula).

Slit-Lamp Examination

A *slit lamp,* or *biomicroscope,* allows the doctor to see signs of infection or disease at the front of the eye, including problems in the eyelids, cornea, *conjunctiva* (the thin, transparent membrane that protects the front of the eye), and iris. Using a higher-powered lens, he or she can also see to the back of the eye, detecting macular degeneration and other problems. During a slit-lamp exam, your head will be comfortably stabilized on the lamp's chin rest.

As its name suggests, the slit lamp shines slits of light into the eye. The size of the slit is adjustable, so the doctor can see very small sections of the eye at very high magnification. The lens nucleus is clearly visible, as are the lens position, the other layers of the lens, and the degree of *brunescence* (browning of the lens), which is responsible for some cataract patients' inability to distinguish blues and purples.

Visual Field Measurement

The simplest way to test your *field of vision*—how far you can see to the left and right out of the corners of your eyes—is for you to focus on the doctor's face while he or she moves a finger slowly to the side and asks you to signal when you can no longer see it. An instrument called a *perimeter,* which emits flashes of light, can be used to reveal *blind spots.* You simply stare at an image and tell the doctor when you see a flash.

Tonometry—Intraocular Pressure (IOP) Measurement

As part of a routine eye exam, your eye doctor will probably use a *tonometer* to screen your eyes for glaucoma. A *noncontact tonometer* is generally used for screening. It expels a puff of air toward the eye and measures the resulting small, instantaneous indentation. The size of the indentation indicates the *intraocular pressure* (IOP) inside the eye. Other types of tonometers are placed directly on the cornea after the eye is numbed with eye drops.

Potential Acuity Testing

If you have cataracts, the doctor may perform *potential acuity testing,* a measure of what your vision would be like if the cataracts were removed. Potential acuity testing is especially useful in determining how much of your vision loss is due to cataracts. One way of testing potential acuity is with a *pinhole acuity meter,* which projects an eye chart directly onto the retina, bypassing the cataract.

Contrast Sensitivity Testing

If cataracts make it hard for you to differentiate shades of gray, you have low *contrast sensitivity.* Your eye doctor might measure this by using a low-contrast visual-acuity chart, or possibly a chart with different contrast levels on symbols of the same size.

Calculating the Power of Your Intraocular Lens

Cataract patients planning to undergo lens-replacement surgery will have tests that examine (a) the power of the cornea and (b) the length of the eye—the primary measurements needed to formulate the synthetic lens to be implanted. The meticulous corneal examinations are also useful for patients with astigmatism and glaucoma.

- *Corneal topography* uses highly sophisticated technology to create a precise three-dimensional map of the cornea.

- *Corneal pachymetry* uses *ultrasound* to measure the thickness of the cornea.

- *Ultrasound biometry ("A-scan")* measures the length of the eye with ultrasound.

- *Optical coherence biometry* also measures the length of the eye but uses light instead of ultrasound.

The ophthalmologist will use all this data to calculate the best *intraocular lens* (IOL) type and power to be implanted. For the most accurate measurements, keep soft contact lenses out of your eyes for three days before your evaluation. If you wear hard contacts or rigid gas permeable (RGP) contacts, stop wearing them three weeks before the evaluation.

Once your cataracts are diagnosed, it will be up to you to decide when they are unacceptably interfering with your work and your lifestyle. The next chapter contains guidelines for the timing of surgery and explains the procedure in detail.

6

Planning for Cataract Surgery

If you're like most people, eventually your cataracts will become more than an inconvenience. Stronger glasses or contacts, magnifying devices and better lighting, and other interim measures can do only so much to help you see better.

When you sense that the time for surgery has come, you'll want to discuss the procedure—removing the natural lens and replacing it with a man-made lens—with your ophthalmologist. Surgery to remove the cataract is the only effective treatment for cataracts, despite promotions you might have seen endorsing cataract-reducing medications, exercises, eye drops, and optical devices.

Cataract surgery produces better vision for nearly all patients—an astounding 98 percent, according to the Eye Surgery Education Council. If you have other eye conditions, such as macular degeneration or advanced glaucoma, your doctor will explain how these disorders might affect the results of cataract surgery and will make treatment recommendations for them.

Are You a Candidate for Cataract Surgery?

Almost anyone who has cataracts and who is in reasonably good health, regardless of age, can have cataract surgery. Here are a few things to keep in mind, however:

- Remember that cataract surgery corrects only cataracts and won't fix other eye problems. Ask your doctor how well you can expect to see after lens replacement if you have macular degeneration, diabetes, glaucoma, extreme nearsightedness, or very small pupils.

- Replacing the clouded lens with a clear one might well improve your eyesight, just as a clear camera lens will give you a sharper photograph than a scratched or blurry lens. But if your retina is damaged, it's like having defective film in your camera. Depending on the type of damage, cataract surgery might or might not help.

- Extremely nearsighted people present special challenges to the surgeon. "High *myopes*" can have excellent results from cataract surgery and lens replacement, but the process is more complicated. They are at greater risk for *retinal detachment,* macular disease, and inflammation than other cataract-surgery patients. It's also harder to calculate the precise "prescription" for the replacement lens and to keep the lens stable after surgery.

Extreme nearsightedness by no means disqualifies you for lens replacement, but you'd be well advised to find an ophthalmologist who is very experienced with cataract surgery on highly myopic patients.

- You'll want to postpone your surgery if you've recently had an infectious (viral or bacterial) illness or any unexplained health problems, such as chest pain.

- If you take blood-thinning medication—aspirin or warfarin (Coumadin), for example—talk with your doctor about the type of surgery you'll be having. You won't have to stop taking blood-thinning drugs if you are having the *clear-corneal phacoemulsification procedure* (described later in this chapter), in which there is no bleeding.

- Don't expect the impossible. In all likelihood, you'll be delighted with the improvement in your eyesight after you've adjusted to your new lenses—as long as you don't expect to see as well as you did in your teens and twenties.

Deciding When to Have Cataract Surgery

Not sure if you're ready for surgery? Here are some of the conditions that might help you make your decision:

- You feel a loss of independence. Perhaps you need help going up and down stairs, or into shops or restaurants, for fear of stumbling, falling, or bumping into things. Glare (from the sun during the day or from headlights at night) might prevent you from driving.

- You can't or don't want to wear glasses or contact lenses.

- Even with eyeglasses or contacts, your vision isn't good enough for you to meet your responsibilities at work, at home, or in the community.

- Vision problems due to cataracts are diminishing your quality of life. If you're an avid reader, photographer, bridge player, or bicyclist, for example, your cataracts might make these pursuits difficult or impossible, or less enjoyable than they could be. They can even be dangerous, if your interests run toward sports and the outdoors: skiing, bicycling, hiking, sailing, and so forth.

Medical factors affecting the timing of cataract surgery include:

- the complexity of surgery and recovery. In general, the longer you wait after cataracts start to bother you, the more complicated the surgery and the longer the recovery.
- health problems, including those affecting your eyes. Cataract surgery is a simple procedure (at least from the patient's perspective) that takes only a few minutes. Still, it's best to have surgery when you are in good health.

Some people don't seek treatment for their cataracts, or they wait until the cataracts are well advanced. They might fear surgery, worry about the length of recovery, or believe that poor eyesight is just "part of getting older."

The fact is, the many benefits of cataract removal and lens replacement greatly outweigh the slight risks. New techniques make the procedure quick and painless; you can have surgery first thing in the morning and be home in time for lunch. Within a few days you can be back at work, already enjoying your clear vision and your independence. You might not need eyeglasses at all, and you can continue to do the things that improve your quality of life. There are benefits for the rest of the population as well. One study has shown that, among people who have cataracts, those who have had cataract surgery are 50 percent less likely to be involved in a car accident while driving.

The Basics of Cataract Surgery

Because virtually everyone eventually develops cataracts, and because cataract surgery is so safe and effective, it is the most common surgical procedure in the United States. Advances in cataract surgery have made the procedure so efficient it can be done in ten to fifteen minutes or less. Recovery is rapid and you might notice dramatic improvements in your vision within a day or two, though the clarity will fluctuate while your eye is healing.

Your doctor will probably operate on one eye at a time, typically doing the procedures a week apart. This way the doctor can make sure that the first eye is healing properly and that there is no infection. The risk of infection is under 1 percent, but if the eye does get infected, your vision could be damaged.

The surgery consists of removing most of the clouded natural lens and replacing it with a clear synthetic lens.

Types of Cataract Surgery

Your doctor will probably remove the clouded lens using *phacoemulsification*, a modern form of *extracapsular cataract surgery*, so called because it leaves much of the lens capsule in place to support the new lens and help with healing.

Phacoemulsification

Phacoemulsification is a process that uses ultra-sound to soften and break apart the clouded lens. The term "phacoemulsification" comes from the Greek *phakos* (referring to the shape of the lens) and the Latin *emulsus* (literally, "milked out"). *Emulsification* is the process of breaking up a substance into fragments that can be suspended in liquid.

In traditional phacoemulsification, the surgeon first injects a local anesthetic behind the eye. For surgery on cataracts in children, in adults who are extremely anxious, and in patients with traumatic eye injury, general anesthesia may be used.

Once the area is numb, the surgeon makes a small incision, removes some of the *anterior* (front) *lens capsule,* and inserts a handheld ultrasonic probe. The probe's high-speed vibration breaks up (emulsifies) the hard nucleus, and an attachment on the probe suctions out the fragments. The lens cortex can be removed by suction alone.

A folded or compressed replacement lens is inserted through the tiny incision. Once inside the eye, the lens unfolds. Then the small incision is closed with only one or two stitches. Traditional phacoemulsification takes about half an hour, with two to three weeks required for recovery.

Clear-Corneal Phacoemulsification

The cataract surgery called clear-corneal phacoemulsification is quickly becoming the procedure of choice among cataract surgeons who want to offer their patients the most effective, least invasive lens extraction and replacement. It is a refinement of traditional phacoemulsification with numerous advantages over the older technique:

- It is painless. The local anesthetic can be administered with eye drops; no needles are used.

- The incision, made with a gem-quality diamond instrument, is only an eighth of an inch long and is so narrow that it is self-sealing, eliminating the need for sutures. Because the incision is placed at the edge of the crystal-clear cornea, there is no bleeding. Eye redness disappears within a day.

- Patients have good vision within a day or two.

- Preexisting astigmatism can be improved and postoperative astigmatism prevented when clear-corneal phacoemulsification is combined with *astigmatism management.* Since astigmatism is caused by irregularities in the shape of the cornea, sometimes the replacement lens itself will correct the astigmatism. *Toric lenses* are used for this purpose.

Otherwise, for astigmatism management, the surgeon might make small incisions in the *limbus*—the thin connection between the cornea and the white of the eye (the sclera). These are called *limbal-relaxing incisions (LRIs),* and they cause the cornea to become more rounded when it heals. Another astigmatism-management technique is to make small incisions of carefully calculated placement and size closer to the center of the cornea. Your surgeon might use a combination of techniques to produce a more-rounded cornea for the best possible surgical results.

Extracapsular Cataract Extraction

Technically, phacoemulsification is a form of extracapsular surgery, since the *posterior capsule* is left in place. In general, however, the term *extracapsular cataract extraction surgery* refers to the method in use before phacoemulsification was developed in the late 1980s. The older method may be preferred by doctors who have been using it for a long time. In rare cases, it is the only solution for patients with multiple eye conditions or with very advanced cataracts that can't be broken up by ultrasound.

After injecting the anesthetic behind the eyeball, the surgeon makes an incision three-eighths of an inch to a half inch long, removes the entire nucleus, and aspirates (suctions out) the cortex. Ten sutures or so are needed to close the incision, which is large

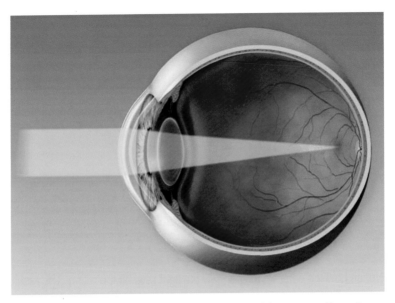

In a normal eye, light passes through the lens and focuses on the retina. Vision is normal.

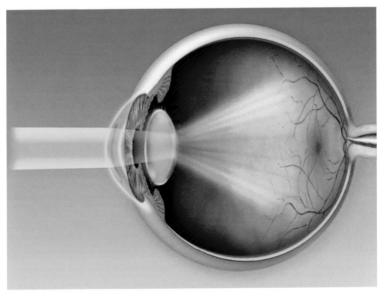

A cataract has formed in the lens of this eye, causing the light rays to scatter rather than focus on the retina. Vision is affected.

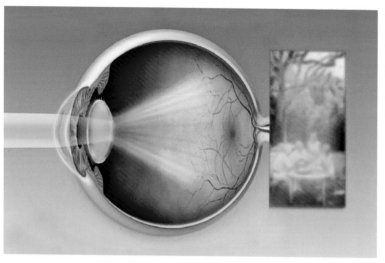

Notice how the cataract affects how the light rays hit the retina. The result is blurred vision.

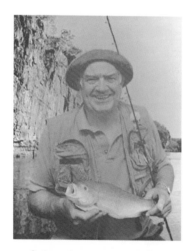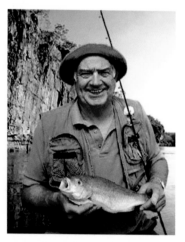

Cataracts can cause color distortion. The photo on the left represents vision with a cataract. The photo on the right represents normal vision.

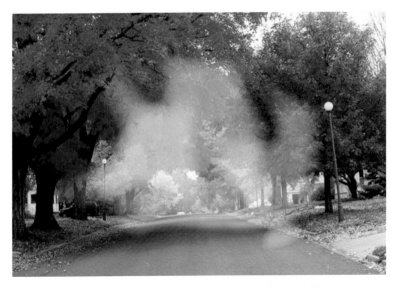

Other symptoms of cataracts are blurry, cloudy, or foggy vision.

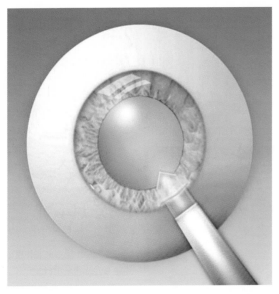

During cataract surgery, a small incision is made in the cornea.

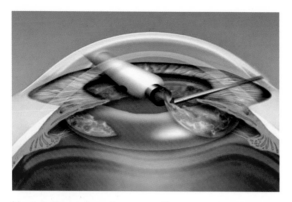

Next during cataract surgery, the surgeon uses an instrument that produces ultrasound waves to break up the lens with the cataract.

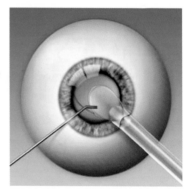

Once the cataract has been removed, the folded intraocular lens is inserted. Once inserted, it unfolds.

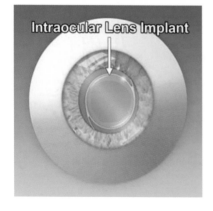

Illustration at the left shows the eyeball with the intraocular lens in place.

enough to accommodate either a foldable replacement lens or a rigid nonfoldable lens.

Full healing takes about eight weeks. As mentioned, the larger incision changes the shape of the cornea and causes or worsens astigmatism. Strong glasses will be needed even after the procedure.

Intracapsular Cataract Extraction Surgery

Intracapsular cataract surgery involves removal of the entire lens, including the capsule. Intracapsular surgery was all but abandoned in the 1980s: It carries more risk and is more painful than extracapsular techniques, and recovery takes much longer. Since there is no remaining capsule to stabilize a replacement lens, patients need to wear thick glasses after this type of surgery.

Refractive Lens Exchange

Refractive lens exchange, simply put, is cataract surgery for someone without visually significant cataracts. Refractive lens exchange can also correct extreme glasses prescriptions that fall outside the range of other surgical techniques such as *LASIK.* Many people with presbyopia, usually in their fifties, choose to have lens-replacement surgery before cataracts have a chance to develop. These people don't want to wear eyeglasses or contacts, and they choose not to have other forms of refractive-error correction, such as LASIK, since within a few years they might well need cataract surgery. With

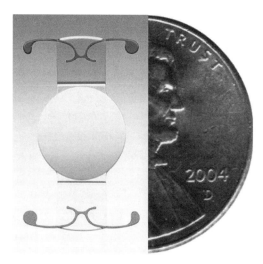

This intraocular lens flexes with the eye's natural muscles, allowing the eye to focus on objects at all distances. The penny shows the size of the IOL.

refractive lens exchange, they are basically killing two birds with one stone—eliminating the need for glasses now and the need for cataract surgery later.

Replacement Lenses

More than 99 percent of cataract surgery patients have intraocular lenses (IOLs) implanted when the natural lenses are removed. Since the cloudy human lens is removed from the eye during cataract surgery, it must be replaced by a man-made lens, the IOL, in order for the eye to recover vision.

Modern IOLs are made of acrylic, silicone, or collagen polymers. They can be rolled or folded to fit through a very small incision. Once inside, they unfold to about a quarter of an inch in size. Side

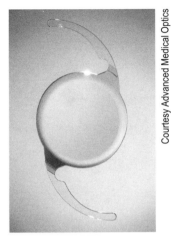

Courtesy Advanced Medical Optics

Shown above is a traditional, single-focus intraocular lens.

struts, called *haptics,* hold them in place within the capsule.

The lens implants become part of the eye. They are safe, stable, and reliable, and they require no care or maintenance other than general practices for good eye health.

Research and development are continually producing IOL refinements: Toric lenses to correct astigmatism, *blue-blocking lenses* to filter out ultraviolet and high-energy blue light, and *aspheric lenses* for better contrast sensitivity are just a few examples.

Intraocular lenses fall into two general categories: *single focus* (standard) and *full focus* (premium). Imagine your range of vision as encompassing five zones, from nearest to farthest. Single-focus lenses provide good vision in only one or two zones, whereas full-focus lenses enable you to see well in three to five zones.

Single-Focus IOLs

A single-focus IOL, also called a *monofocal IOL*—like a disposable camera lens—has a single fixed focal point, usually designed for mid-distance vision, so you'll need eyeglasses to see near objects and those farther than arm's length. Still, your vision will be better at some distances than it was before surgery.

If you don't mind wearing glasses, monofocal lenses might work well for you. If you choose the standard single-focus IOL, you should be prepared to wear glasses for many or most activities.

This multifocal intraocular lens provides a wide range of vision, both near and distant. The "bulls-eye" rings in the lens make this possible.

Full-Focus IOLs

Full-focus IOLs are more like high-end Nikon camera lenses, automatically adjusting their focus to provide good near, mid-range, and distance vision without glasses. Many patients who choose full-focus IOLs can do almost anything they wish without glasses. Manufacturers of full-focus lenses use different technologies in the production of lenses.

Full-Focus Multifocal IOLs

Multifocal IOLs have different focusing zones built into the lens, allowing a wide range of vision with decreased dependence on glasses. Since these IOLs work by dividing the light that enters the eye, they can produce glare and halos, particularly at night.

Full-Focus Accommodating Lenses

Most IOLs, once implanted, remain in a fixed position within the lens capsule. *Accommodating lenses,* also called *adaptive lenses,* respond to contracting and loosening of the ciliary muscles, moving within the eye for smooth accommodation through the entire range of vision. The ciliary muscle changes the shape of the synthetic lens, just as it did with the natural lens while it was still flexible, before the onset of presbyopia.

Though your vision will be better immediately after implantation of an adaptive lens, it can take up to a year for the ciliary muscle to get used to the new lens. During that time, you'll experience slight fluctuations in clarity of vision.

Monovision

Monovision refers to implanting IOLs in different strengths, making one eye more distance-dominant and the other eye more near-dominant. If the implants are premium accommodating IOLs, a wide range of sharp vision without glasses is possible.

If you've successfully worn monofocal contact lenses, you might be a good candidate for monovision. The brain usually adapts to the difference in *refraction.* Very seldom are the results unsatisfactory, requiring corrective LASIK. If you and your doctor are considering monovision for your lens implants, he or she might want you to try wearing monofocal contact lenses for a while before your surgery.

Piggyback Lenses

If you have had cataract surgery and you're not satisfied with the results, it's possible to implant new lenses on top of the existing ones. This process is called *piggybacking*. It can't correct every type of damage, and the best option is to choose your surgeon carefully so that the procedure will be done right the first time.

7

Your Cataract Procedure

Your eye surgeon will give you specific instructions to follow before and after your procedure and will tell you what to expect during the procedure. The following guidelines apply to clear-corneal phacoemulsification, which is easier on the patient than other types of cataract surgery. Even for the same procedure, however, the routine can vary greatly from clinic to clinic and from doctor to doctor. If what you read in the paragraphs below differs from your doctor's instructions, *follow your doctor's instructions.*

Before Surgery

Preoperative Consultation

If you haven't already done so, take with you to the consultation your medical history, family medical history, and a record of drugs and supplements you use or have recently used. It's a good idea to ask your spouse or partner or a friend to go to the consultation with you.

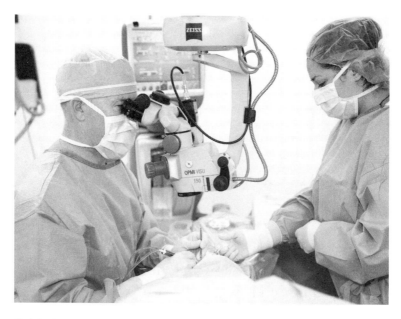

Ophthalmologists use a microscope to perform cataract surgery. The procedure usually takes about ten minutes per eye to perform.

To select the right type of replacement lens, your doctor will want to know about your work and other responsibilities, your hobbies and interests, and any other activities that are meaningful to you. Be prepared to tell the doctor how you feel about wearing eyeglasses occasionally, often, or all the time, and whether near, mid-range, or distant vision is most important to you.

Preoperative Health Evaluation

Your eye doctor will probably want your internist or primary-care physician to do a physical examination and lab work within a month or so before your surgery. The purpose is to verify that you are healthy enough to have the surgery, that you're not having unexplained symptoms such as chest pain, and that you haven't had a recent cough, cold, or flu episode.

Preoperative Instructions

Three days before surgery. Start using the antibiotic eye drops your surgeon has prescribed. If you wear contact lenses, remove the lens from the eye to be treated and leave it out. If you haven't yet done so, arrange for someone to drive you home after surgery. This is important, because you will *not* be able to drive right after surgery: You'll be a little

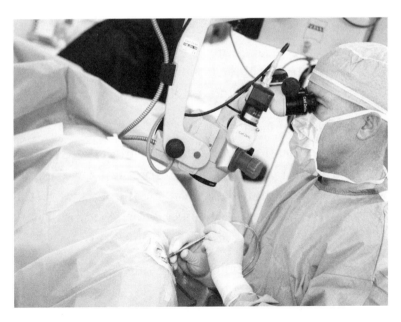

During cataract surgery, the eye surgeon inserts the foldable intraocular lens through an incision measuring less than one-eighth inch.

73

groggy from the sedative, your pupil will be dilated, and your eye may still be "asleep."

The day before surgery. Don't have anything to eat or drink for the eight hours preceding your surgery. You can take necessary medications with a small amount of water.

The day of surgery. Don't wear makeup or fragrances, including scented lotions or hair products. Don't take or wear jewelry or other valuables. Do wear comfortable street clothes, including a shirt that buttons up the front. These are the clothes you'll be wearing during surgery, so make sure they're loose, not binding.

- Do take your medications and insurance card to the surgical center.
- Do arrive an hour before the scheduled time for surgery. Plan to be at the surgical center for about two and a half hours.

At the Surgical Center

A fully staffed operating room in a certified surgical center is the best environment for cataract surgery. High standards for cleanliness and the presence of a board-certified anesthesiologist can help ensure that there are no complications.

- Nursing staff will check your blood pressure and insert an intravenous (IV) line, which the anesthesiologist will use to administer a mild sedative.

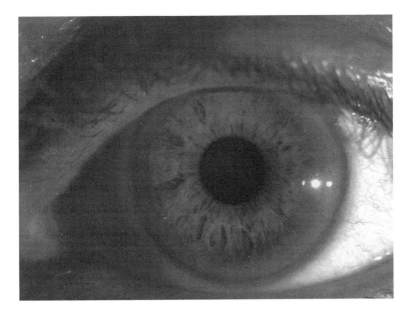

This eye is shown after cataract surgery. The IOL is not visible—it sits behind the iris of the eye.

- About thirty minutes before the surgery, a nurse will put drops in your eye to numb the area and to dilate the pupil.

- In the operating room, your eyelid, eye-lashes, and face will be cleaned with an anti-bacterial iodine solution. Your doctor will want to eliminate any possibility of infection. The iodine cleansing is just one of several ways of ensuring that the procedure is completely sanitary.

- After giving you a sedative through the IV line, the anesthesiologist will place small heart monitors at the top of your chest. (This is why it's recommended that you wear a front-buttoning shirt.) The sedative won't put you to sleep; you'll be awake but relaxed during surgery.

- You'll lie on your back, completely covered with a special sterile sheet that has an opening over the eye. The rest of your face will be covered to keep bacteria from your nose and mouth away from your eye.

- A small tube, similar to a drinking straw, will be placed beneath the sheet on your chest. During the time your face is covered, this tube will release a gentle flow of oxygen toward your face.

The anesthesiologist will be sitting by your side the entire time, monitoring your vital signs throughout the procedure.

During the Procedure

The actual procedure—clear-corneal phacoemulsification and synthetic-lens implantation—can take as little as five minutes. Clear-corneal phacoemulsification is painless. At first, all you'll feel is the surgeon's hand resting against your cheek.

Patients sometimes ask if they will see the surgery being performed. The answer is no. You might see bright lights or kaleidoscopic colors, as in a light show, but the experience won't be unpleasant.

- After the doctor makes a tiny incision at the edge of the cornea, using a gem-quality diamond instrument, he or she will put more anesthetic into the eye. No needles are used in clear-corneal phacoemulsification.

- As described, the doctor will use a handheld ultrasound device to break up the hard nucleus and suction out the fragments and the lens cortex, leaving the posterior capsule in place to support the new lens. At this stage you might feel a few drops of cool water running down your face. The water is used during surgery to keep the eye cool.

- The new lens, or IOL, is inserted. After inserting the lens, the doctor will administer more eye drops—additional anesthetic, antibiotic, and anti-inflammatory medication—for your comfort and safety.

After Surgery

In the recovery room, a nurse will check your blood pressure again, give you something to eat or drink, and monitor you for a half hour to an hour or so. Then you can go home and take a nap. You'll receive special sunglasses to wear on the way home, since your pupil will be dilated and highly sensitive to bright light.

It will take an hour or so for your eye to recover from the anesthetic drops. During this time, it's normal for the affected eye to see only black and possibly a few shadows. When your vision returns, it will be blurry but will gradually improve over the course of the day.

At home, use the prescribed eye drops as instructed, first washing your hands thoroughly with regular soap. You probably won't have any discomfort at all. Most patients don't even need Tylenol, but it's okay to take an over-the-counter pain pill if you're slightly uncomfortable.

By evening, if you're rested and your vision allows, go out for dinner with friends. They'll be amazed that there's no redness or puffiness in the eye that was operated on and that you can already see well enough to be out and about. You'll go to the doctor's office for a short follow-up visit the day after surgery. Your vision will be fairly good, but, to be on the safe side, have someone drive you to and from the appointment.

Guidelines for Care at Home

Once you've seen the doctor in your next-day follow-up visit, you can go home and relax for another day or two, *or* go back to your normal routine right away, with a few exceptions:

- For the first few days, don't wear eye makeup. If you use mascara, buy a fresh tube to use when you start wearing eye makeup again. The fresher your cosmetics, the less likely they are to contain harmful bacteria.

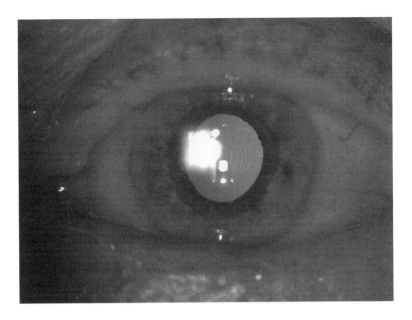

This photo was taken after the insertion of an IOL. Vision usually returns within hours after the surgery. In most cases, vision is good the next day and excellent in about a week.

- For one week, avoid heavy lifting (more than fifty pounds) and other strenuous activities that might elevate your blood pressure.

- It's okay to resume moderate exercise after a few days, but avoid breath holding (as when lifting weights, since holding your breath can raise your eye pressure) and jarring activities (such as running on concrete) for several days. If you're a workout buff, ask your ophthalmologist what forms of exercise are safe and how soon you can resume your full routine.

- Continue to use the antibiotic and anti-inflammatory eye drops until your doctor says it's okay to stop—usually a few weeks after surgery.
- Stay out of swimming pools, hot tubs, Jacuzzis, steam baths, and saunas for two weeks. Showering and bathing are fine.
- Avoid rubbing your eye for four weeks.

Vision Immediately after Surgery

Don't be surprised if your vision fluctuates for several days as the eye heals and the pupil returns to its normal size. Your eyesight might seem to be getting worse, then better, off and on for a few weeks. As mentioned, you'll notice fluctuations in your vision for a few weeks or even longer if you have had an accommodating lens implanted. This is normal and expected.

Inside the eye there will be swelling and inflammation. These symptoms should subside within a week, but each patient is different. Younger patients, in their fifties or sixties, and those with milder cataracts, heal more quickly than patients who are older or whose cataracts were extensive. Be assured, however, that the amount of time it takes your eye to heal won't change the ultimate outcome.

You'll see everything more clearly—including any preexisting *floaters,* those little objects in the vitreous humor that float across your field of vision.

So if occasionally you notice something that looks like a gnat hovering at the edge of your field of vision, it's nothing to be concerned about.

Results of Cataract Surgery

After your eyes have healed and your brain and muscles have adjusted to the implanted lenses, your world will be brighter and clearer. You'll be able to focus better. Objects won't appear distorted—*ghosting* and double vision, though possibly not eliminated completely, will no longer be a problem. Colors will appear richer and more distinct. Contrast will be sharper.

You'll see well enough to work, to move around independently, and to enjoy the activities that you might have put on hold. You'll be less dependent on eyeglasses—you might not need them at all. Ideally, you'll be able to read the newspaper in good light. You probably won't be able to read the tiny print on products such as sweetener packets without a magnifying glass, but that's okay. Cataract surgery isn't a fountain of youth, but it does improve your vision. Being in your sixties, seventies, eighties, or nineties, and having the vision of a forty-year-old, is an amazing thing in itself.

As mentioned, your vision will fluctuate for a few weeks or longer, depending on the type of lens implanted. Even so, within twenty-four hours your eyesight will be markedly improved—so much so that you'll probably be eager to schedule surgery for the other eye at your follow-up visit to your doctor.

Cataract surgery is a low-risk procedure, and complications are rare. Still, you should be aware of possible side effects and potential problems, which are discussed in the next chapter.

8

Risks and Side Effects of Cataract Surgery

The success of your surgery is greatly dependent on the skill and experience of your surgeon. It's important that you make a careful, informed choice regarding your surgeon and that you follow his or her instructions for aftercare, including follow-up visits.

No replacement lens, however sophisticated it might be, is as good as a young, healthy, crystal-clear natural lens. Though your vision will almost certainly be better than before your surgery, it will not be as sharp as a teenager's. Nighttime halos and glare, double vision, and ghosting might not be eliminated altogether.

Even so, by replacing a clouded natural lens—which is only going to get worse over time—with a clear, durable, state-of-the-art synthetic lens, you will see images more vividly than you have for years (including those occasional dots in your field of vision—tiny fragments known as floaters). You'll enjoy greater independence and a wider range of activities. And all this will be possible with less dependence—maybe even *no* dependence—on eyeglasses.

Normal Side Effects

For a few days after your cataract surgery you might experience a slight aching or tenderness of the eye. Only about 5 percent of patients are uncomfortable enough to take an over-the-counter pain reliever. Also normal and to be expected are itching, scratchiness, watering or dryness, and sensitivity to light.

As mentioned, you'll notice fluctuations in your vision for a few weeks or even longer, depending on the lens implanted and your own healing process. These changes should not be severe enough to interfere with your day-to-day activities.

Potential Complications During Surgery

In the clear-corneal phacoemulsification procedure, the incision is minuscule and no needles are used, making complications during surgery relatively rare. Complications such as rupture of the capsule, perforation of the eye, bleeding from the *choroid,* and damage to a nerve were much more common in past years, when cataract surgery was more invasive.

Retained Cataract Fragments

Very rarely, fragments of the cataract fall into the vitreous cavity, the space between the lens and the retina, and may have to be removed surgically to prevent inflammation.

Potential Complications After Surgery

Complications from cataract surgery occur in only a tiny percentage of patients. The risks are almost nil in the hands of an excellent surgeon. When rare complications do occur, however, a few can be serious and might require immediate medical attention.

Be sure to ask your doctor what you should do—both during and after office hours—if you have symptoms of potentially serious complications.

Infection

Fewer than one-tenth of 1 percent (0.1%) of cataract-surgery patients get *endophthalmitis*, a bacterial (or occasionally fungal) infection of the inner eye. Symptoms can include pain, loss of vision, and excessive redness. If not treated immediately, the condition might damage the vision. The usual treatment is injection of antibiotics into the eye. Rarely, *vitrectomy*—removal of the vitreous—is necessary to control the infection.

Retinal Detachment

In about one-half of 1 percent (0.5%) of patients, vitreous fluid seeps through a tear in the retina after cataract surgery, separating the retina from the back of the eye. Extremely nearsighted patients are at greater-than-normal risk for retinal detachment.

Symptoms include a shower of new floaters, much like a swarm of bees, in the vision, or extensive flashes of light, akin to fireworks. The most distinctive symptom is complete or partial loss of vision in the affected eye. Patients report feeling as if a curtain is moving across their field of vision.

Like infection, retinal detachment is a medical emergency. If you have symptoms of either, you should seek treatment immediately, day or night.

Inflammation

Slight inflammation within the eye is normal for a day or two after surgery. Very unusual is prolonged inflammation of eye membranes (*uveitis*) or the macula (*cystoid macular edema*, caused by accumulation of fluid in the retina). These can usually be managed using anti-inflammatory eye drops. *Corneal edema*, an inflammation of the cornea, may in extreme cases require a cornea transplant. Report any eye pain, tenderness, or swelling to your ophthalmologist immediately.

Lens Shifting

Rarely, the implanted lens shifts or rotates within the eye. It can be replaced surgically, although wearing thin eyeglasses usually solves the problem.

Incorrect Prescription

A capable, experienced eye surgeon will carefully formulate the prescription for your lens using measurements of the cornea and the length of the eye. This formulation is more difficult if you are extremely farsighted or nearsighted or if you've had LASIK or another type of *refractive surgery*—all of which underscores the importance of finding the best ophthalmologist available, ideally one who specializes in cataract surgery. If it turns out that the lens is too strong or too weak, the solution is to perform additional surgery to improve the focusing or rarely to replace it surgically.

After-Cataract (Secondary Cataract)

When the clouded natural lens is removed and a synthetic lens implanted, it's impossible for cataracts to "come back." Sometimes, however, the natural lens capsule, part of which remains in the eye to hold the implanted lens in place, becomes clouded or thickened. This posterior capsule opacity—which can develop months or years after your surgery—is also called an *after-cataract* or *secondary cataract*. It is quite common and affects younger patients more often than older patients.

Fortunately, the problem can be quickly and safely repaired with a five-minute outpatient procedure called *YAG laser capsulotomy.* Your eye surgeon will use an *yttrium aluminum garnet (YAG) laser* to make a small hole in the back of the lens capsule, allowing light through. The procedure is painless, requiring no incision or sutures.

When to Call Your Doctor

Get in touch with your doctor right away or follow his or her emergency instructions if you are concerned about symptoms that are more severe or last longer than expected. These may include inflammation (pain, redness, swelling), haziness, marked decrease in vision, nausea, vomiting, excessive coughing, light flashes, or multiple floaters.

9

The Future of
Cataract Treatment

As baby boomers approach their mid-sixties, the volume of cataract surgery is skyrocketing, as is the demand for even greater safety, convenience, and visual acuity. Accordingly, researchers throughout the world are investigating, testing, or introducing lens materials, surgical techniques, and prevention methods that could revolutionize the treatment of not only cataracts but also other eye conditions, such as glaucoma, macular degeneration, and presbyopia. Here is just a sample of cataract-related scientific work in various stages of development:

Cataract Prevention Strategies

- Formulation of chemical compounds to prevent or halt cataract development, which might also stop the progression of muscular dystrophy, traumatic brain injury, and Type 2 diabetes

- The use of topical antioxidants to remove heavy metal ions from the eye, with promising results, especially in the treatment of diabetic cataracts
- Genetic research that could lead to gene therapy for cataracts and other eye disorders

Prevention of After-Cataracts (Posterior Capsule Opacification)

- Improvements in IOL design and materials, such as development of a polyethylene glycol coating that would prevent formation of opacities on the capsule
- Refinements in phacoemulsification techniques

Intraocular Lens (IOL) Improvements

- Development of an implantable lens gel
- Development of IOLs whose focusing strength can be adjusted after cataract surgery by applying the appropriate wavelength of light to change the lens's shape

Also Being Studied

- Development of IOL injection devices, combined with new ultrasonic probes, for use in incisions as small as one millimeter

- Refinements in IOL power calculation
- Prevention of infection and inflammation by implanting a drug-delivery device in the eye
- A two-stage cataract procedure, consisting of standard cataract surgery followed by refractive surgery using a special laser to precisely adjust the shape of the cornea
- Presbyopic corneal inlays, for improved near vision while retaining distance vision

Ophthalmic researchers and optical scientists envision exciting possibilities for safe, noninvasive ways to prevent and correct vision damage in people of all ages. Some of the developments described above are many years away from practical application. Others are just becoming available for use by experienced and highly skilled eye surgeons.

One thing is certain: Cataract surgery and lens replacement have made huge strides in just the past few years. The procedure is safer and faster, and the results more satisfying, than anyone could have imagined in the days when, after cataract surgery, patients had to wear thick, heavy eyeglasses to have any vision at all. If you have cataract surgery today, and your surgeon has kept abreast of improved techniques and materials, you can thank the pioneering work of scientists and eye specialists for restored clarity of vision, independence, and quality of life that you will appreciate as never before.

Resources

American Academy of Ophthalmology
P.O. Box 7424
San Francisco, CA 94120-7424
Phone: 415-561-8500
Fax: 415-561-8533
www.aao.org

American Foundation for the Blind
11 Penn Plaza, Suite 300
New York, NY 10001
Phone: 212-502-7600
Toll-free: 800-AFB-LINE (232-5463)
E-mail: afbinfo@afb.net
www.afb.org

American Optometric Association
243 North Lindbergh Boulevard
St. Louis, MO 63141
Phone: 314-991-4100
Toll-free: 800-365-2219
www.aoa.org
Washington-area office
1505 Prince Street, Suite 300

Alexandria, VA 22314
Phone (toll-free): 800-365-2219
www.aoa.org

American Society of Cataract and Refractive Surgery Eye Surgery Education Council
4000 Legato Road, Suite 700
Fairfax, VA 22033
Phone: 703-591-2220
www.ascrs.org
www.eyesurgeryeducation.com

The Foundation of the American Academy of Ophthalmology
P.O. Box 429098
San Francisco, CA 94142-9098
Phone: 415-561-8500
www.eyecareamerica.org

National Eye Institute
U.S. National Institutes of Health
2020 Vision Place Bethesda, MD 20892-3655
Phone: 301-496-5248
www.nei.nih.gov
www.nei.nih.gov/health/cataract/
    cataract_facts.asp

Prevent Blindness America
Vision Health Resource Center
211 West Wacker Drive, Suite 1700
Chicago, IL 60606
Phone: (toll free) 800-331-2020
www.preventblindness.org
www.diabetes-sight.org

Glossary

20/20 vision: Normal visual acuity. The numbers indicate that the tested eye, twenty feet away from the eye chart, sees as well as a "normal" eye at the same distance.

Ablation: Removal, or vaporization, of tissue with a laser.

Accommodating intraocular lens: A type of intraocular lens (IOL) that enables the patient to focus automatically, via "retraining" of the ciliary muscle and zonules, at a range of distances in much the same way as with a clear, flexible natural lens.

Accommodation: The eye's ability to change lens shape (by action of the ciliary muscle and zonules) in order to focus clearly on objects at various distances. As the lens becomes more rigid with age—a condition called presbyopia—it is less able to accommodate.

Adaptive intraocular lens: See *accommodating intraocular lens.*

Aftercataract: Opacity that develops on the posterior lens capsule after extracapsular cataract removal.

Amblyopia: Poor vision, usually in one eye but occasionally in both eyes, that develops between birth and age six. Caused by continued suppression of vision in the affected eye, not by structural abnormality.

Amsler grid: Grid consisting of lines on contrasting background (black on white or white on black) used to test for macular degeneration or other central-visual-field defects.

Anterior chamber: Area between the cornea and the iris filled with aqueous humor.

Antioxidant: Molecule or compound, such as vitamins C and E and selenium, that can bond with and neutralize free radicals, preventing cell damage.

Aphakia: Absence of the crystalline lens of the eye.

Aqueous, aqueous humor: Clear, watery fluid that fills the anterior chamber of the eye; maintains intraocular pressure and nourishes the cornea, iris, and lens.

A-scan: Ultrasound device used to distinguish normal from abnormal eye tissue or to measure eye length.

Aspheric intraocular lens: A type of IOL that is slightly flattened around the edges; believed to offer better contrast sensitivity than traditional IOLs, on which the front surface is curved.

Astigmatism: Visual distortion caused by a cornea whose surface is elongated—like the side of a football—rather than curved like an arc on a sphere. Light rays enter the eye unequally and may produce two focal points on the retina.

Astigmatism management: A surgical procedure designed to prevent or minimize worsening of astigmatism, a common side effect of cataract surgery.

Autorefractor: A device, used to test refractive error, that emits a pinpoint beam of light, which reflects off the retina and measures the eye's response.

Best corrected visual acuity (BCVA): The best vision possible with corrective lenses.

Bioavailability: The ease with which a nutrient is absorbed and used by the body.

Biological age: A person's age measured by the condition of the muscles, brain, lungs, and sensory organs, unlike chronological age, measured in calendar years.

Biomicroscope: See *slit lamp.*

Blind spot: Sightless area within normal visual field; caused by absence or blockage of light-sensitive photoreceptors on the retina (specifically the fovea).

Blue-blocking intraocular lens: An IOL that filters out high-energy blue light, which can damage the retina and contribute to macular degeneration.

Blunt cannula: A narrow tube with a blunted tip, designed to perform many of the piercing functions of a surgical needle but without the needle stick.

Brunescence: Browning of the crystalline lens due to cataracts.

Capsule: A thin membrane that forms the outermost layer of the crystalline lens, above the cortex and the nucleus.

Cataract: Clouded area (opacity) of the crystalline lens; caused by trauma, disease, or aging, or may be congenital.

Central vision: In the visual field, the area of sharpest vision, used for reading and distinguishing detail and color. See also *peripheral vision.*

Choroid: Layer of blood vessels that provide oxygen and nutrients to the retina.

Ciliary body: Eye structure that contains ciliary muscle, which contracts or relaxes, thereby changing the shape of the crystalline lens and allowing it to focus on objects at varying distances.

Ciliary muscle: See *ciliary body*.

Clear-corneal phacoemulsification: An advanced type of cataract surgery in which the incision is placed at the edge of the clear cornea. Clear-corneal phacoemulsification does not require the use of needles, does not cause bleeding, uses a very small (one-eighth of an inch or smaller) incision, and allows for rapid recovery.

Color blindness: Inability to clearly distinguish certain colors. So-called red-green color blindness is usually hereditary. Yellowing of cataracts can also cause a degree of color blindness.

Cone: One of more than 7 million retinal photoreceptor cells (in each eye) concentrated in the macular area (specifically the fovea centralis) of the retina, responsible for sharp vision and ability to see colors.

Congenital cataract: A cataract that is present at birth.

Conjunctiva: Clear mucous membrane that covers the white of the eye (sclera) and lines the inner surface of the eyelids.

Contrast sensitivity: Ability to visually distinguish dark objects against a light-colored background, or light-colored objects against a dark background.

Cornea: Clear, curved protrusion at the front of the eye through which light first passes; provides 70 percent of the eye's focusing power. The cornea covers and protects the iris, pupil, and anterior chamber.

Corneal edema: Abnormal fluid buildup and consequent swelling of the cornea.

Corneal pachymetry: Measurement of corneal thickness using ultrasound.

Corneal topography: Rendering of a precise three-dimensional map of the cornea using sophisticated camera and computer technology.

Cortex: Soft, clear tissue that forms the middle layer of the crystalline lens, between the capsule and the nucleus.

Cortical cataract: A cataract that begins as whitish, wedge-shaped opaque areas on the outer edge of the lens cortex, near the capsule, eventually becoming streaks reaching inward to the center of the lens, like spokes on a wheel.

Cosmic radiation: Atomic radiation that bombards Earth from outer space. Earth's atmosphere provides protection from these harmful rays, which can cause cataracts in airline pilots and astronauts.

Cover test: Part of an eye examination, often used to detect strabismus or amblyopia. While the patient looks directly at an object, the eye doctor covers one eye and quickly notes how much the uncovered eye moves to adjust.

Cross-eye: See *esotropia.*

Crystalline lens: The eye's natural lens; a flexible, transparent tissue, located behind the iris, that helps focus rays of light onto the retina.

Cystoid macular edema: A condition in which fluid-filled cysts develop in the macula, causing retinal swelling.

Diabetes mellitus: A group of diseases that develop when the body is unable to use blood sugar for energy, causing excessive amounts of sugar in the bloodstream (hyperglycemia).

Dilation: Enlargement (of an opening). With reference to the eye, dilation of the pupil occurs naturally in dim light, allowing more of the available light into the eye. Eye doctors also chemically dilate the pupil during an eye examination in order to have a better view into the interior of the eye.

Diopter: A measurement of refractive error—a positive number in the case of hyperopia (farsightedness), and a negative number to describe myopia (nearsightedness).

Diplopia: See *double vision.*

Double vision: A type of distortion in which two images of a single object are seen. Common with cataracts and other eye disorders.

Emmetropes: People who have no refractive error; that is, no nearsightedness, farsightedness, or astigmatism. Perfect refractive ability is referred to as *emmetropia.*

Endophthalmitis: A serious infection, usually bacterial, of the interior of the eye.

Epithelium: The cornea's outermost layer of cells, forming the eye's first defense against infection.

Esotropia: Lack of coordination between eye movements in which one eye is normally aligned and the other is aligned inward. Also called "cross-eye." See also *strabismus.*

Excimer laser: A "cold" laser, so called because it can remove corneal tissue without heating it during refractive surgery.

Exotropia: Lack of coordination between eye movements in which one eye is normally aligned and the other is aligned outward. Also called "wall-eyes."

Extracapsular cataract surgery: A form of cataract surgery, such as phacoemulsification, that leaves much of the lens capsule in place to support the new lens and help with healing. The term also refers to the more-invasive extracapsular procedure that was common before phacoemulsification, involving a larger incision, removal of the intact nucleus, approximately ten sutures, and an extended recovery period.

Eyelid: Thin, retractable tissue covering the front of the eye. The eyelid serves to protect the eye from dust and other foreign objects and from exceedingly bright light. It also distributes moisture (tears) over the cornea.

Farsightedness: See *hyperopia.*

Field of vision: See *visual field.*

Floaters: Particles in the vitreous humor that drift across the visual field.

Folding intraocular lens: An IOL that can be inserted through a tiny incision by being folded or rolled; it then opens to normal size within the eye.

Fovea, fovea centralis: Central concave area of the macula that is packed with photoreceptors called cones, which produce the sharpest vision.

Free electron: The unpaired electron in a free radical.

Free radical: An atom, usually oxygen, that has an odd number of electrons, leaving one electron unpaired and making the atom unstable.

Fundus: Interior surface of the back of the eyeball, visible with an ophthalmoscope. The eye's fundus includes the retina (with macula and fovea) and the juncture of the optic nerve with the eye.

Ghost images: Distortion of vision similar to "seeing double." With double vision, however, you'll see two relatively clear images, whereas ghost images are fainter "copies" that appear on one side of or around the object you're looking at.

Ghosting: A type of image distortion, fairly common with cataracts. See also *ghost images.*

Glare: Sensation of dazzling, intense, scattered light when looking at light source; often due to cataracts.

Glassblower's cataract: A cataract that is caused by infrared (heat) radiation, usually as a result of occupational exposure, as in the case of arc welders and glassblowers.

Glaucoma: Group of diseases usually associated with increased intraocular pressure; if untreated, can lead to blindness.

Gonioscope: Device used to examine the eye's anterior chamber, using a magnifier and mirror-equipped contact lens.

Halo: Perceived rings around light sources viewed at night; often accompanied by glare. A common symptom of cataracts.

Haptics: The side struts, or extensions, on an intraocular lens that help to hold it in place after implantation.

Hypermature cataract: A cataract that is so far advanced it may be completely opaque and allow little or no vision in the affected eye; can cause pain and inflammation.

Hyperopia: Farsightedness, occurring when the eye is "too short" and images come into focus behind the retina. A farsighted person, or *hyperope*, may see well at a distance but have trouble with near vision.

Immature cataract: A cataract that is not well advanced, cannot be seen with the naked eye, and may not yet interfere significantly with vision.

Intracapsular cataract surgery: A type of cataract surgery, rarely used today, that involves removal of the entire lens, including the capsule.

Intraocular lens: A synthetic lens implanted during cataract surgery to replace the natural lens.

Intraocular pressure (IOP): Fluid pressure within the eye.

IOL: See *intraocular lens.*

Iris: The colored ring in the visible eye. Contracts or recedes around the pupil to regulate the amount of light that enters the eye.

Keratotomy: A surgical incision of the cornea.

Laser: Acronym for *light amplification by stimulated emission of radiation,* a high-energy light source used medically to cut, burn, or dissolve tissues.

LASIK: Acronym for *laser assisted in situ keratomileusis,* a refractive-surgical procedure to reshape the cornea and change its optical power.

Lazy eye: See *amblyopia.*

Legal blindness: Best corrected visual acuity of 20/200 or worse.

Lens: See *crystalline lens.*

Limbal-relaxing incisions: An astigmatism-management technique consisting of small incisions in the limbus—the thin connection between the cornea and the white of the eye (the sclera)—that cause the cornea to become more rounded when it heals.

Low vision: Poor visual acuity.

Macula: Small central area of the retina filled with light-sensitive photoreceptors called rods and cones.

Macular degeneration: A progressive eye disease caused by deterioration of the central portion of the retina, called the macula.

Mature cataract: A cataract that has advanced to the point where the lens appears milky.

Monofocal intraocular lens: An IOL that is similar to a disposable camera lens, in that it has a single fixed focal point, usually designed for mid-distance vision. Eyeglasses are needed for good vision at other distances.

Monovision: Adjustment, using corrective lenses or surgery, of one eye for near vision and the other for distance vision.

Multifocal intraocular lens: An IOL that is similar to a sophisticated camera lens, in that it automatically adjusts its focus to provide good near, mid-range, and distance vision without glasses.

Myopia: Nearsightedness, occurring when the eye is "too long" and images come into focus before they reach the retina. A nearsighted person, or myope, may have good near vision but have difficulty seeing objects at a distance.

Nearsightedness: See *myopia.*

Noncontact tonometry: A method of measuring intraocular pressure (that is, pressure of fluids within the eye) in which the testing instrument does not come in contact with the cornea.

Nuclear cataract: Clouding of the center of the lens (nucleus), almost always due to aging.

Nucleus: The firm center, or core, of the crystalline lens, surrounded by the cortex, which in turn is inside the capsule.

Ophthalmologist: A medical doctor who specializes in the diagnosis and medical or surgical treatment of eye disorders and disease.

Ophthalmoscope: An illuminated instrument using mirrors to examine structures in the back of the eye.

Optic nerve: Bundle of nerve fibers that transmit visual impulses from the retina to the brain.

Optical coherence biometry: Measurement of eye length using light, rather than ultrasound as in an A-scan.

Optician: One who is trained to fit and dispense eyeglasses and, in some U.S. states, contact lenses, according to a prescription from an optometrist or ophthalmologist. Outside the United States, some countries license ophthalmic opticians to do eye exams.

Optometrist: A doctor of optometry (O.D.), qualified to diagnose and treat vision disorders not requiring specialized medical or surgical intervention.

Orbit: The bony socket that surrounds the eyeball.

Overripe cataract: See *hypermature cataract.*

Pachymetry: Measurement of corneal thickness.

Perimeter: A device that emits flashes of light to test field of vision and reveal blind spots.

Peripheral vision: Side vision; in the visual field, perception of objects outside the direct line of vision. See also *central vision.*

Phacoemulsification: Surgical procedure to remove a cataract using ultrasound to break up the lens, which is then removed by suction.

Phoropter: An eye-examination device consisting of a complete range of corrective lenses that can be adjusted to hundreds of combinations, which the patient is asked to evaluate. By continually changing the lenses, the doctor can arrive at a combination of lens strengths that becomes the basis of a prescription for corrective lenses.

Photoreceptor cells: Light-sensitive cells—rods and cones—on the retina that allow the eye to see in dim light, distinguish colors, and perceive contrast.

Piggyback intraocular lens: An IOL that is implanted on top of an existing IOL.

Pinhole acuity meter: Projection of an eye chart directly onto the retina, bypassing the lens, used to test potential acuity.

Posterior capsular opacification: Aftercataract; an opacity that can develop on the posterior capsule at any time after lens replacement.

Posterior capsule: The rear part of the lens capsule, which is left in place during cataract surgery to help support the implanted lens.

Posterior chamber: The fluid-filled area between the iris and the lens.

Posterior subcapsular cataract: A cataract that begins at the back of the lens, just under the lens capsule.

Potential acuity: A presurgical assessment of a patient's likely visual acuity if cataracts were removed.

Presbyopia: Loss of sharpness in near vision caused by age-related stiffening of the crystalline lens and accompanying reduction in ability to accommodate.

Pupil: Black circular opening in the center of the iris. Through muscular action of the iris, the pupil shrinks or grows (dilates) to regulate the amount of light that enters the eye.

Refraction: Bending of light as it passes from one material to another. Also, a test to determine the eye's refractive error.

Refractive error: Optical defect producing blurred vision due to light rays not converging precisely on the retina; nearsightedness, farsightedness, or astigmatism.

Refractive lens exchange: Like cataract surgery, a procedure to remove the crystalline lens and replace it with a synthetic lens. Refractive lens exchange, however, is performed before cataracts have developed significantly, generally because the patient cannot or does not wish to wear eyeglasses or contact lenses.

Refractive surgery: Procedure to correct refractive error, often by changing the shape of the cornea.

Retina: Smooth, thin layer of tissue, at the back of the eye, containing photoreceptor cells, which convert reflected light into electrical impulses that move along the optic nerve to the brain.

Retinal detachment: Separation of the retina from the underlying pigment epithelium, requiring immediate surgery to prevent blindness.

Retinal pigment epithelium: The part of the retina consisting of dark tissue cells that absorb excess light and carry nutrients to, and waste products from, the retina.

Ripe cataract: See *mature cataract.*

Rod: One of more than 120 million retinal photoreceptor cells (in each eye) that are especially receptive to brightness and allow us to see in dim light.

Sclera: The "white of the eye"; an opaque, fibrous, protective covering that surrounds the eye.

Second sight: A temporary, cataract-induced improvement in vision among nearsighted people.

Secondary cataract: See *aftercataract.*

Slit lamp: A microscope that projects a flattened beam of light into the eye for close examination of internal structures.

Snellen's chart: Standard assessment instrument for visual acuity; chart consisting of rows of letters (largest at the top, smallest at the bottom) developed by Dutch ophthalmologist Hermann Snellen in 1862; usually read at a distance of twenty feet.

Socket: The protective bony cavity that holds the eyeball.

Steroid: A drug, often a type of hormone, that is used medically to relieve swelling and inflammation.

Strabismus: Eye misalignment caused by imbalance in muscles that hold the eyeballs; often referred to as "cross-eye."

Subcapsular cataract: See *posterior subcapsular cataract.*

Tear: Thin film of fluid that lubricates the front of the eye. Blinking spreads tear film evenly across the surface.

Tonometer: An instrument, often used in glaucoma testing, that measures pressure of fluids inside the eye.

Tonometry: Measurement of intraocular pressure.

Toric intraocular lens: An IOL specially designed to correct astigmatism.

Traumatic cataract: A cataract that is caused by direct eye injury, head injury near the eye, earlier eye surgery, eye inflammation, chemical burns, or electric shock. Some scientists consider radiation a form of "slow trauma" that contributes to cataract development.

Tunic: One of three layers of the eyeball that surround the fluid-filled center.

Ultrasound: High-energy sound waves, often projected onto internal structures, creating echoes of different magnitudes that can be visualized on a television screen.

Ultrasound biometry: See *A-scan*.

Ultraviolet radiation (UV): Electromagnetic radiation, shorter in wavelength than visible radiation but longer than X-rays; invisible rays of the sun responsible for damage to skin and eyes.

Uvea, uveal tract: Eye layer between retina and sclera that contains the iris, ciliary body, and choroid.

Uveitis: Inflammation of the uvea.

Visual acuity: Sharpness of vision.

Visual field: Extent of the area visible to an eye looking straight ahead; includes central and peripheral vision.

Vitrectomy: Surgical removal of the vitreous, which is replaced with clear fluid.

Vitreous, vitreous humor: Clear gel-like substance that fills the rear two-thirds of the eyeball, between the lens and the retina.

Wall-eyes: See *exotropia.*

YAG laser: Yttrium aluminum garnet laser, which produces a short-pulse, high-energy light beam to cut or perforate tissue.

Zonule: One of the fibers that connect the ciliary muscle to the crystalline lens. Contraction and relaxation of the ciliary muscle change the tension of the fibers, which in turn changes the focusing power of the eye. The fibers also help to hold the lens in place.

Index

20/20 vision, 7, 48

A

A-scan, 54
accommodating lenses, 69
accommodation, 12
acuity, 47
adaptive lenses, 69
after-cataract, 87, 88
    prevention, 90
aftercare, 83
age-related cataracts, 24
    mature, 24
    ripe, 24
aging
    as a risk factor, 34–38
air pollution, 34
alcohol abuse, 35
Alzheimer's disease, 34
amblyopia, 47
American Academy of
    Ophthalmology, 45
American Foundation for
    the Blind, 30
anesthesiologist, 74–76
anterior chamber, 5
anterior lens capsule, 62
anti-inflammatory
    medication, 77, 80, 86

antibiotic eye drops, 73, 77,
    80
antibiotics, 85
antioxidants, 36
    foods, 36–38
    fruits, 37, 38
    other sources, 37, 38
    vegetables, 37
arc welding, 40
aspheric lenses, 67
aspirin, 58
astigmatism, 14–16, 47, 54
    correction, 67
    management, 63, 64
    preexisting, 63
autorefractor, 50

B

bacteria, 8, 76, 78
bacterial infection, 85
baseline eye exam, 45
bioavailability, 36
bioflavonoids, 36
biological age, 33
biomicroscope, 52
bleeding, 63
blind spots, 52
blinding sensation, 11
blindness and cataracts, 25,
    26

About Dr. Maloney

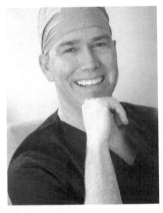

Robert K. Maloney, **MD, MA (Oxon)**, is an ophthalmologist and a cataract and LASIK specialist in Los Angeles, California, where he is Director of the Maloney Vision Institute. Dr. Maloney has personally performed more than 50,000 eye surgeries.

He specializes in providing optimum vision without glasses using laser and cataract surgery. He is a former Rhodes Scholar and Summa Cum Laude graduate of Harvard University; he completed his education at Oxford University and Johns Hopkins Hospital. Dr. Maloney is also Clinical Professor of Ophthalmology at UCLA. He was voted by his peers as one of America's top ten vision-correction specialists in a nationwide survey conducted by *Ophthalmology Times*.

He is the recipient of the prestigious 2001 Distinguished Lans Award, given annually to one surgeon in the world for innovative contributions to the field of vision correction surgery. The American Academy of Ophthalmology awarded him the Senior Honor Award for contributions to the education of other eye surgeons and the Secretariat Award for contributions to the Academy. Dr. Maloney is also co-author of *LASIK—A Guide to Laser Vision Correction*, and he has published more than 100 articles, abstracts, and reports in professional journals and has delivered more than 200 invited lectures on five continents.

Dr. Maloney's research is focused on developing new surgical techniques, including the implantable contact lens and the light-adjustable lens implant for cataract surgery. He developed the "Maloney Method," a widely used way of calculating lens implant power for cataract surgery in patients with prior LASIK surgery. He has been a principal investigator for fifteen FDA clinical trials. Dr. Maloney has appeared frequently on television as the eye surgeon for the ABC hit series *Extreme Makeover.* He has been interviewed by the Discovery Channel, The Learning Channel, NBC's Extra, ABC's *20/20* and *Prime Time Live*, PBS's *Life and Times*, and CNN's *The World Today*.

Dr. Maloney may be reached by calling the Maloney Vision Institute at 877 EYESIGHT, or 310-208-3937; or he may be reached through his Web site: **www.maloneyvision.com**.

Consumer Health Titles from Addicus Books

Visit our online catalog at www.addicusbooks.com

Straight Talk about Breast Cancer—
 From Diagnosis to Recovery $19.95
The Stroke Recovery Book—
 A Guide for Patients and Families $19.95
The Surgery Handbook—
 A Guide to Understanding Your Operation $14.95
Understanding Lumpectomy—
 A Treatment Guide for Breast Cancer $19.95
Understanding Parkinson's Disease, 2nd Edition $19.95
Understanding Peyronie's Disease $16.95
Understanding Your Living Will $12.95
Your Complete Guide to Breast Augmentation
 & Body Contouring $21.95
Your Complete Guide to Breast Reduction & Breast Lifts . $21.95
Your Complete Guide to Facial Cosmetic Surgery $19.95
Your Complete Guide to Facelifts $21.95
Your Complete Guide to Nose Reshaping. $21.95

To Order Books:

Visit us online at: www.addicusbooks.com

Call toll free: 800-352-2873

For discounts on bulk purchases,
call our Special Sales Dept. at (402) 330-7493

Book Order Form

Please send:

_____copies of _____

at_____each.

Total   _____

Nebraska residents add 6.5% sales tax   _____

Shipping/Handling   _____

$5.00 postage for first book: _____

$1.20 for each additional book: _____

TOTAL ENCLOSED   _____

Name _____

Address_____

City _____State _____Zip _____

☐ Visa ☐ MasterCard ☐ American Express ☐ Discover

Credit card number _____

Expiration date _____

Ways to Order:

- Mail order by credit card, personal check, or money order.
  Send to: Addicus Books, P.O. Box 45327, Omaha, NE 68145

- **Order TOLL FREE:** 800-352-2873

- **Visit us online at:** www.addicusbooks.com

- **For discounts on bulk purchases, call our Special Sales Dept. at
  402-330-7493**